Pathology

PreTest®
Self-Assessment
and Review

Pathology

PreTest® Self-Assessment and Review

Seventh Edition

Edited by

Margaret H. S. Clements, M.D.
Visiting Professor of Pathology
Cornell University Medical College
New York, New York

With questions contributed by

Michael D. Jeffers, M.B.
Senior House Officer
St. James's Hospital
Dublin, Ireland

McGraw-Hill, Inc.
Health Professions Division/PreTest Series

New York   St. Louis   San Francisco   Auckland
Bogotá   Caracas   Lisbon   London   Madrid
Mexico   Milan   Montreal   New Delhi   Paris
San Juan   Singapore   Sydney   Tokyo   Toronto

Pathology: PreTest® Self-Assessment and Review, Seventh Edition
Copyright © 1993 1991 1988 1986 1983 1980 1976 by McGraw-Hill, Inc. All rights
reserved. Printed in the United States of America. Except as permitted under the
Copyright Act of 1976, no part of this publication may be reproduced or distributed
in any form or by any means, or stored in a data base or retrieval system, without
the prior written permission of the publisher.

1 2 3 4 5 6 7 8 9 0   DOCDOC   9 8 7 6 5 4 3 2

ISBN 0-07-051999-4

The editors were Gail Gavert and Bruce MacGregor.
The production supervisor was Gyl A. Favours.
This book was set in Times Roman by Compset, Inc.
R.R. Donnelley & Sons was printer and binder.

Library of Congress Cataloging-in-Publication Data

Pathology : PreTest self-assessment and review.—7th ed. /
    edited by Margaret H. S. Clements ; with questions
    contributed by Michael D. Jeffers.
        p.   cm.—(Basic sciences series)
    Includes bibliographical references.
    ISBN 0-07-051999-4
    1. Pathology—Examinations, questions, etc.
    I. Clements, Margaret H. S.   II. Jeffers, Michael D.
    [DNLM: 1. Pathology—examination questions.
    QZ 18 P297]
    RB31.P325   1993
    616.07′076—dc20
    DNLM/DLC
    for Library of Congress   91-38986
                                                               CIP

Contents

Preface

The study of pathology, a science so basic to clinical medicine, has been abbreviated sadly in many medical schools in recent years, and this at a time when explosive growth is occurring in the science. Recent advances in immunopathology, diagnosis of bacterial and viral diseases including AIDS, and detection of infectious agents such as papillomavirus in cervical dysplasia are proceeding at a tremendous rate. The seventh edition of *Pathology: PreTest® Self-Assessment and Review* includes such new subject areas as predictive values in the interpretation of laboratory data, importance of cytokines, the molecular basis of genetic and other disease processes, and molecular biology techniques as these apply to lymphoproliferative disorders and other tumors.

The medical student must feel submerged at times in the flood of information—occasionally instructors may have similar feelings. This edition is not intended to cover all new knowledge in addition to including older anatomic and clinical pathology. It is, rather, a serious attempt to present important facts about many disease processes in hopes that the student will read much further in major textbooks and journals and will receive some assistance in passing medical school, licensure, or board examinations.

Introduction

Pathology: PreTest® Self-Assessment and Review provides medical students, as well as physicians, with a comprehensive and convenient instrument for self-assessment and review within the field of pathology. The 500 questions parallel the same format and degree of difficulty of the questions contained in Step 1 of the United States Medical Licensing Examination (USMLE) as well as the Foreign Medical Graduate Examination in the Medical Sciences (FMGEMS).

To conform with current USMLE guidelines, all K-type (multiple true-false) questions have been eliminated.

Each question in the book is accompanied by an answer, an explanation, and specific page references to current textbooks, journal articles, or both. A bibliography, listing all the sources used, follows the last chapter.

Perhaps the most effective way to use this book is to allow yourself one minute to answer each question in a given chapter; as you proceed, indicate your answer beside each question. By following this suggestion, you will be approximating the time limits imposed by the board examinations previously mentioned.

When you finish answering the questions in a chapter, you should then spend as much time as you need verifying your answers and carefully reading the explanations. Although you should pay special attention to the explanations for the questions you answered incorrectly, you should read *every* explanation. The author of this book has designed the explanations to reinforce and supplement the information tested by the questions. If, after reading the explanations for a given chapter, you feel you need still more information about the material covered, you should consult and study the references indicated.

Pathology

**PreTest®
Self-Assessment
and Review**

General Pathology

DIRECTIONS: Each question below contains five suggested responses. Select the **one best** response to each question.

1. Which of the following provides an example of concomitant hyperplasia and hypertrophy?

(A) Uterine growth during pregnancy
(B) Left ventricular cardiac hypertrophy
(C) Enlargement of skeletal muscle in athletes
(D) Breast enlargement at puberty
(E) Cystic hyperplasia of the endometrium

2. Type I collagen is found in all the following EXCEPT

(A) tendon
(B) dermis
(C) cartilage
(D) fascia
(E) bone

3. Which group of factors is most important in the cellular pathogenesis of acute ischemia?

(A) Mitochondrial hyperplasia, lysozyme release, membrane injury
(B) Reduced ATP, increased calcium influx, membrane injury
(C) Lipid deposition, reduced protein synthesis, nuclear damage
(D) Ribosome detachment, glycolysis, nuclear damage
(E) Mitochondrial condensation, glycolysis, sodium cell loss

4. During early inflammation following margination of leukocytes, an important adhesive surface protein on leukocytes is

(A) interleukin 1 (IL-1)
(B) complement factor 5a (C5a)
(C) endothelial leukocyte adhesion molecule (ELAM-1)
(D) tumor necrosis factor (TNF)
(E) leukocyte function antigen 1 (LFA-1)

1

5.   A very important mediator of the systemic effects of inflammation is

(A) gamma interferon (γ-IFN)
(B) beta tumor necrosis factor (β-TNF)
(C) interleukin 1 (IL-1)
(D) interleukin 2 (IL-2)
(E) interleukin 3 (IL-3)

6.   Defects in chemotaxis resulting in increased susceptibility to infection are associated with all the following EXCEPT

(A) diabetes mellitus, juvenile type
(B) chronic granulomatous disease of childhood
(C) chronic renal failure of any cause
(D) Chédiak-Higashi syndrome
(E) newborn infants of normal gestation

---

7.   The cluster of cells in the photomicrograph below appeared in a cytologic specimen of sputum from a 57-year-old man with chest pain, hemoptysis, and a nonproductive cough of many years' duration. Which of the following is the most likely diagnosis?

(A) Squamous cell metaplasia of ciliated, bronchial epithelium
(B) Oat cell (small cell undifferentiated) carcinoma
(C) Adenocarcinoma
(D) Cytomegalic inclusion virus pneumonia
(E) Normal bronchial epithelium

8. An understanding of complex disorders like hereditary spherocytosis, Chédiak-Higashi syndrome, and alcoholic liver disease has improved with molecular discoveries in

(A) lysosomal release
(B) recombinant DNA
(C) cytoskeletal makeup
(D) membrane phospholipids
(E) lipid accumulation

9. Endotoxic shock is commonly caused by all the following organisms EXCEPT

(A) *Pseudomonas aeruginosa*
(B) *Escherichia coli*
(C) *Proteus* species
(D) *Corynebacterium diphtheriae*
(E) *Klebsiella pneumoniae*

---

10. The cells in the photomicrograph shown below are from a drop of cerebrospinal fluid. The most likely diagnosis is

(A) subarachnoid hemorrhage
(B) viral meningitis
(C) tuberculous meningitis
(D) bacterial meningitis
(E) leukemic meningitis

11. The chemical mediators of inflammation listed below often proceed in a cascade after activation EXCEPT

(A) complement
(B) kinin
(C) arachidonic acid
(D) fibrinopeptides
(E) neutral proteases

12. Carcinoma of the oral cavity

(A) is predominantly adenocarcinoma in type
(B) is more common in females
(C) is predisposed to by hairy leukoplakia
(D) is predisposed to by erythroplasia
(E) occurs most frequently on the hard palate

13. The photomicrograph below of a duodenal aspiration smear shows an organism that

(A) is often numerous in lymph nodes
(B) infects principally the large intestine
(C) is transmitted by the genus *Triatoma*
(D) is the most common intestinal parasite in the U.S.
(E) is frequently identified in cervicovaginal smears

14. All the following characteristics are true of liposarcoma EXCEPT that it

(A) presents varied histology
(B) is commonly found in the retro-peritoneum
(C) frequently gives rise to emboli-zation in lymphatics
(D) is the most common soft tissue sarcoma
(E) arises very rarely in subcuta-neous tissue

15. The cells of the mononuclear phagocyte system originate from the

(A) spleen
(B) liver
(C) lymph node
(D) bone marrow
(E) thymus

16. The histologic pattern of the lymph node section shown below is likely to support a diagnosis of

(A) sickle cell anemia
(B) carcinoma
(C) leukemia
(D) infectious mononucleosis
(E) rheumatoid arthritis

17. In tissues affected by the predominant form of Niemann-Pick disease, which of the following is found at abnormally high levels?

(A) Sphingomyelin
(B) Sphingomyelinase
(C) Kerasin
(D) Acetyl coenzyme A
(E) Ganglioside

18. The diseases of the Hand-Schüller-Christian complex all involve the

(A) skeleton
(B) reticuloendothelial system
(C) heart
(D) lungs
(E) teeth and nails

19. All the following symptoms are associated with Klinefelter's syndrome EXCEPT

(A) large, soft testes
(B) gynecomastia
(C) eunuchoidism
(D) azospermia
(E) elevated urinary gonadotropins

20. If a mutant gene is not expressed phenotypically in a person, this is said to represent

(A) variable expressivity
(B) reduced penetrance
(C) codominance
(D) genetic heterogeneity
(E) nondisjunction

21. Fibrosarcoma, shown in the photomicrograph below, may be characterized by all the following EXCEPT

(A) interlacing bundles of anaplastic spindle cells
(B) occasional similarity to "cellular fibroma"
(C) fibroblastic or myofibroblastic differentiation
(D) relative infrequency of occurrence
(E) association with hyperglycemia

22. A 23-year-old man with full-blown AIDS is noted to be severely neutropenic. Which of the following abnormalities is most likely to be seen on further investigation?

(A) Macrocytic anemia
(B) Normal CD4 lymphocyte count
(C) Thrombocytopenia
(D) Eosinopenia
(E) Hypocellular bone marrow

23. In an evaluation of an 8-year-old boy who had had recurrent infections since the first year of life, findings included enlargement of the liver and spleen, lymph node inflammation, and a superficial dermatitis resembling eczema. Microscopic examination of a series of peripheral blood smears taken during the course of a staphylococcal infection indicated that the bactericidal capacity of the boy's neutrophils was impaired or absent. Which of the following is the most probable diagnosis?

(A) Chronic granulomatous disease
(B) Congenital agammaglobulinemia
(C) Hereditary thymic dysplasia
(D) Chédiak-Higashi syndrome
(E) Wiskott-Aldrich syndrome

24. The irregular eosinophilic hyaline inclusions within the hepato-cytoplasm shown below are

(A) Russell bodies
(B) parasites
(C) characteristic of chronic alcoholism
(D) characteristic of viral hepatitis
(E) characteristic of carbon tetrachloride poisoning

25. Interest is growing in recently discovered cell markers on neoplastic cells that are designated

(A) ADCC
(B) A1AT
(C) HIV-1
(D) TSTA
(E) ARC

26. All the following cytologic and membrane alterations can generally be found in neoplastic cells EXCEPT

(A) changes in pseudopodia and microvilli
(B) changes in the cytoskeleton
(C) acquisition of surface-associated glycoproteins
(D) increased lectin agglutinability
(E) decreased membrane transport

27. The cells seen in the following photomicrograph were stained by ABC technique using OKT1 (Leu-1), OKT3 (Leu-4), and OKT11 (Leu-5) cluster designation CD5, CD3, and CD2. The result indicates that the cells are of what origin?

(A) T lymphocytes
(B) Oat cells
(C) Mesothelial cells
(D) EAC rosettes
(E) Melanoma cells

28. Natural killer (NK) cells have all the following characteristics EXCEPT

(A) the ability to lyse virus-infected cells
(B) cytoplasmic granules containing myeloperoxidase
(C) increased activity with stimulation by IL-2 and interferon
(D) the ability to function without prior sensitization
(E) NK receptors and Fc receptors for IgG

CMC

29. After receiving incompatible blood, a patient develops a transfusion reaction in the form of back pain, fever, shortness of breath, and hematuria. This type of immunologic reaction is classified as a

(A) systemic anaphylactic reaction
(B) systemic immune complex reaction
(C) delayed-type hypersensitivity reaction
(D) complement-mediated cytotoxicity
(E) T cell–mediated cytotoxicity

30. An industrial foundry worker who has been chronically exposed to heavy metal vapors has developed a radiographic pattern of pulmonary "honeycombing." Which of the following heavy metals is most likely responsible?

(A) Cobalt
(B) Lead
(C) Cadmium
(D) Mercury
(E) Arsenic

31. An allograft is a graft between

(A) a human and an animal
(B) two individuals of different species
(C) two individuals of the same species
(D) two individuals of the same inbred strain
(E) identical twins

32. Which of the following conditions is most likely to be associated with cancer?

(A) Systemic lupus erythematosus
(B) Hypertension
(C) Polymyositis
(D) Autoimmune thyroiditis
(E) Arteriosclerosis

33. True statements concerning diagnostic specificity include all the following EXCEPT

(A) Scl-70 antibody is specific for diffuse systemic sclerosis
(B) antibodies to nucleolar RNA are specific for diffuse systemic sclerosis
(C) antibodies to double-stranded DNA are specific for systemic lupus erythematosus (SLE)
(D) antibodies to antinuclear antibody (ANA) are specific for SLE
(E) anti-Sm antibodies are specific for SLE

34. Systemic lupus erythematosus (SLE), a multisystem disease of autoimmune origin, is characterized by all the following statements EXCEPT

(A) polyclonal B-cell activation is essential to the pathogenesis
(B) membranous glomerulonephritis is the most common renal lesion
(C) visceral lesions are mediated by type III hypersensitivity
(D) joint involvement (arthritis) is common clinically
(E) hypergammaglobulinemia is usual

35. All the following statements regarding primary Sjögren's syndrome are true EXCEPT

(A) xerostomia is a major symptom
(B) anti-SSB antibodies are major markers
(C) renal glomerular lesions are common
(D) rheumatoid factor is often present
(E) there is increased frequency of HLA-DR3

---

36. A patient with severe diabetic renal disease receives a donor cadaver kidney, following which a progressive rise in the serum creatinine occurs over a period lasting 5 months. In the photomicrograph below, what single finding is most characteristic for chronic rejection?

(A) Damaged glomeruli
(B) Interstitial fibrosis
(C) Interstitial inflammation
(D) Tubular atrophy
(E) Vascular changes

37. An adult patient in the summer months suffers a rash on one of the extremities followed several weeks later by arthritis of the knee. In addition to viral and bacterial disorders and rheumatoid joint disease, which of the following should also be considered in the differential diagnosis?

(A) Hemarthrosis
(B) Reiter's disease
(C) Lyme disease
(D) Charcot's joint
(E) Baker's cyst

38. Hypertrophic osteoarthropathy is most often associated with

(A) bronchiectasis
(B) infective endocarditis
(C) bronchogenic carcinoma
(D) mesothelioma
(E) inflammatory bowel disease

39. Using an immunofluorescent procedure for detection of serum antibodies to mitochondria, one would expect a negative result in

(A) primary biliary cirrhosis
(B) chlorpromazine-induced jaundice
(C) acute viral hepatitis
(D) chronic active hepatitis
(E) systemic lupus erythematosus

40. A young woman of average intelligence and short stature who has never menstruated is under clinical investigation for Turner's syndrome. However, a buccal smear shows some cells having one Barr body. Which of the following best explains this finding?

(A) Laboratory error
(B) The patient is a male
(C) Classic XO pattern
(D) Turner's mosaic pattern
(E) Klinefelter's syndrome

41. Normal levels of C-reactive protein (CRP) are most often observed in

(A) acute viral illness
(B) pneumococcal pneumonia
(C) active rheumatoid arthritis
(D) active pulmonary tuberculosis
(E) acute myocardial infarction

42. The most specific of the commonly used tests for diagnosing active syphilis is the

(A) rapid plasma reagin (RPR) test
(B) *Treponema pallidum* immobilization (TPI) test
(C) fluorescent treponemal antibody-absorption (FTA-ABS) test
(D) Venereal Disease Research Laboratory (VDRL) test
(E) Kolmer test

43. Characteristic features of lepromatous leprosy include all the following EXCEPT

(A) nerve involvement
(B) numerous bacilli in histiocytes
(C) frequent polyclonal hypergammaglobulinemia
(D) association with erythema nodosum
(E) encroachment of infiltrate on basal epidermis

44. As visualized by the electron microscope, all the following are cell organelles EXCEPT

(A) lysosomes
(B) the Golgi complex
(C) the endoplasmic reticulum
(D) desmosomes
(E) microbodies

45. Spirochetal infections include all the following EXCEPT

(A) bejel
(B) yaws
(C) relapsing fever
(D) Weil's disease
(E) lymphogranuloma venereum

46. An elevated IgG level in cerebrospinal fluid and an abnormal band on agar gel electrophoresis of cerebrospinal fluid are findings consistent with the diagnosis of

(A) secondary stage of syphilis
(B) muscular dystrophy
(C) tumor involvement of the spinal cord
(D) meningeal involvement by leukemia
(E) multiple sclerosis

47. In hemolytic disease of the newborn, all the following statements are correct EXCEPT

(A) erythroblastosis fetalis develops because of prior maternal sensitization
(B) anemia and hepatosplenomegaly are characteristic
(C) anti-D immunoglobulin should be given to a sensitized mother before delivery
(D) both ABO and Rh antigens cause hemolytic disease of the newborn
(E) there is transplacental transmission of maternal antibody

48. The gross texture and resilience of a given tumor are largely influenced by which of the following?

(A) Presence or absence of connective tissue stroma
(B) Degree of malignancy
(C) Interface between normal tissue and tumor
(D) Type of epithelium present
(E) Relative blood supply

49. A 37-year-old woman who has a clinical picture of fever, splenomegaly, varying neurologic manifestations, and purplish ecchymoses of the skin is found to have a hemoglobin level of 10.0 g/dL, a mean corpuscular hemoglobin concentration (MCHC) of 48, peripheral blood polychromasia with stippled macrocytes, and spherocytes, with a blood urea nitrogen level of 68 mg/dL. The findings of coagulation studies and the patient's fibrin-degraded products are not overtly abnormal. Which of the following is most closely identified with these findings?

(A) Idiopathic thrombocytopenic purpura
(B) Thrombotic thrombocytopenic purpura
(C) Disseminated intravascular coagulopathy
(D) Submassive hepatic necrosis
(E) Waterhouse-Friderichsen syndrome

50. The "stat" laboratory sends the following electrolyte results to the ward concerning a new admission: Na^+, 142 meq/L; K^+, 7.2 meq/L; Cl^-, 101 meq/L; and CO_2, 32 meq/L. On the basis of these results, the physician should

(A) treat with sodium exchange resin
(B) institute peritoneal dialysis immediately
(C) inquire about a hemolyzed blood sample
(D) infuse insulin intravenously
(E) make a diagnosis of hyperkalemia

51. Parathyroid hormone, by its action on target organs, is known to cause all the following EXCEPT

(A) increased intestinal calcium absorption
(B) increased renal tubular reabsorption of calcium
(C) increased serum phosphate levels
(D) mobilization of calcium from bone
(E) decreased renal tubular reabsorption of phosphate

52. The enzyme activity curve labeled II, shown below, best represents the pattern for which of the following serum enzymes after an uncomplicated acute myocardial infarction?

(A) Glutamic-oxaloacetic transaminase
(B) Creatine phosphokinase
(C) Lactic dehydrogenase
(D) Alkaline phosphatase
(E) 5'-Nucleotidase

53. A 65-year-old known diabetic man is admitted with fever, dehydration, and altered consciousness, with no perceptible odor of acetone on his breath. The serum Na^+ level is 146 meq/L, the glucose level is 960 mg/dL, and the blood urea nitrogen (BUN) level is 48 mg/dL. Calculate the serum osmolality.

(A) 280 mosmol
(B) 310 mosmol
(C) 318 mosmol
(D) 356 mosmol
(E) Insufficient data

54. Elevated levels of serum amylase are found in all the following conditions EXCEPT

(A) morphine administration
(B) diabetic ketoacidosis
(C) mumps
(D) renal insufficiency
(E) congestive heart failure

55. Which of the following assays is the most reliable and cost-effective screening method in separating Cushing's syndrome from conditions with similar features, such as obesity?

(A) Urinary 17-ketosteroids
(B) Urinary 17-ketogenic steroids
(C) Urinary 17-hydroxysteroids
(D) Urinary free cortisol
(E) Plasma cortisol

56. Elevated levels of serum alkaline phosphatase are expected findings in each of the following conditions EXCEPT

(A) obstructive jaundice
(B) cirrhosis
(C) pregnancy (last trimester)
(D) polycythemia vera
(E) hepatitis

57. What is the creatinine clearance of a person who passes 361 mg of creatinine in a 24-h urine sample of 770 mL and whose plasma creatinine is 2.0 mg/100 mL (2.0 mg/dL)?

(A) 12.5 mL/min
(B) 25.0 mL/min
(C) 50.0 mL/min
(D) 75.0 mL/min
(E) 100.0 mL/min

58. Hyperuricemia often occurs secondary to all the following disorders EXCEPT

(A) myeloproliferative disorders
(B) carcinoma
(C) chondrocalcinosis (pseudogout)
(D) starvation
(E) chronic renal disease

59. A 20-year-old student has an upper respiratory infection with severe sore throat and pain on swallowing. Her dormitory roommates make a diagnosis of infectious mononucleosis, thus saving her a trip to the student health center. Six weeks later, she develops a low-grade fever and back pain. A urinalysis finding of red blood cell casts

(A) reflects glomerular damage
(B) is insignificant if few casts are present
(C) is probably due to a menstrual "contaminant"
(D) suggests the presence of hemorrhagic cystitis
(E) is present in any instance of hematuria

60. While many factors affect a tumor's behavior, which of the following can be expected to influence the biology of a given tumor the *most*?

(A) Lack of a peripheral capsule
(B) Histologic differentiation
(C) Presence of inflammation
(D) Size of the tumor
(E) Nuclear cytoplasmic ratio

61. Pathogenic pneumococci typically exhibit all the following EXCEPT

(A) inhibition of growth by ethylhydrocupreine (Optochin)
(B) M protein in their cell walls
(C) bile solubility
(D) positive Neufeld quellung reactions
(E) detection of capsular polysaccharides by counterimmunoelectrophoresis (CIE)

62. An adult patient suffers from recurrent bleeding from the gums, intermittent GI bleeding, and excessive bleeding from minor trauma to the skin. A prolonged bleeding time is discovered. Which of the following levels or activities should be assessed to complete the diagnosis?

(A) Prothrombin time
(B) Plasma fibrinogen
(C) Factor VIII:R
(D) Factor VIII:C
(E) Factor VIII:Ag

63. The table below shows the normal serum values for the five isoenzymes of lactic dehydrogenase (LDH) and the values obtained for one patient. The diagnosis most compatible with the patient's values is

Isoenzyme	Normal % activity	Patient's % activity
LDH$_1$	20–35	18
LDH$_2$	30–40	24
LDH$_3$	20–30	13
LDH$_4$	5–15	26
LDH$_5$	1–15	19

(A) acute hepatitis
(B) pernicious anemia
(C) pulmonary infarct
(D) myocardial infarct
(E) cerebrovascular accident

64. An African boy with a rapidly expanding mass in the region of the jaw and cheek is thought to have Burkitt's lymphoma. These cells are growing rapidly because of

(A) their permanent nature
(B) shortening of the cell cycle
(C) nonsequencing of the EBV genome
(D) fewer G_0 cells entering the cycle
(E) delayed progression from G_2 to mitosis

65. Environmental and industrial pollutants are becoming increasingly relevant in human oncogenesis. Which of the following combinations is most closely allied with human neoplasia?

(A) Asbestos, silica, arsenicals
(B) Diethylstilbestrol, radioactive dusts, cyanide
(C) Aflatoxin, beryllium vapor, benzidine
(D) Polyvinyl chloride, nickel, chromium
(E) Carbon tetrachloride, lead, chloroform

66. Which of the following is physiologically the most active thyroid hormone?

(A) Thyroglobulin
(B) Monoiodotyrosine (MIT)
(C) Diiodotyrosine (DIT)
(D) Triiodothyronine (T_3)
(E) Thyroxine (T_4)

67. A diagnosis of adrenogenital syndrome with demonstrable adrenal hyperplasia is consistent with

(A) generalized calcium oxalate deposition similar to that occurring in oxalosis
(B) accumulation of glycolipids in tissues
(C) salt loss simulating Addison's disease
(D) symptoms similar to those occurring in phenylketonuria
(E) severe acidosis

68. True statements regarding celiac disease (nontropical sprue) include that

(A) there is a strong association with HLA-B8 and HLA-Dw3 antigens
(B) severity of disease often correlates strongly with serum level of antibody to gliadin
(C) malignancy is unassociated
(D) many of the mucosal inflammatory cells express surface IgG antigliadin
(E) the distal small bowel shows the most severe involvement

69. All the following genetic disorders are autosomal recessive (AR) EXCEPT

(A) alkaptonuria
(B) familial hypercholesterolemia
(C) phenylketonuria (PKU)
(D) myeloperoxidase deficiency
(E) cystic fibrosis (CF)

70. A chromosomal aberration that results in a disturbance in the normal gene balance is termed

(A) nondisjunction
(B) euploidy
(C) aneuploidy
(D) breakage
(E) variance

71. The major underlying defect in classical renal tubular acidosis (caused by gradient defect) appears to be

(A) an excessive back-diffusion of secreted hydrogen ions from tubular urine to blood
(B) an impairment of ammonia excretion
(C) a leakage of bicarbonate ions out of the proximal tubule
(D) a deficiency in the total hydrogen ion secretory capacity
(E) an impairment in the reclamation of filtered bicarbonate ions

72. Lobar pneumonia is caused predominantly by

(A) *Klebsiella pneumoniae*
(B) *Staphylococcus pyogenes*
(C) *Haemophilus influenzae*
(D) *Streptococcus pneumoniae*
(E) *Legionella pneumophila*

73. The most common type of disordered porphyrin metabolism (porphyria) is

(A) intermittent acute porphyria
(B) variegate porphyria
(C) protoporphyria
(D) congenital erythropoietic porphyria
(E) porphyria cutanea tarda

74. Characteristically, B lymphocytes do all the following EXCEPT

(A) constitute 10 to 15 percent of peripheral blood lymphocytes
(B) occur in lymphoid follicles and the superficial cortex of lymph nodes
(C) express surface immunoglobulins IgM and IgD
(D) express cluster differentiation antigen CD8
(E) possess complement component (C3) receptors

75. Which of the following organisms produces signs and symptoms that mimic acute appendicitis?

(A) Enteropathic *Escherichia coli*
(B) *Enterobius vermicularis*
(C) *Trichomonas hominis*
(D) *Yersinia enterocolitica*
(E) *Bacillus anthracis*

76. Delayed-type hypersensitivity reactions of the tuberculin skin test type

(A) appear within 1 or 2 h
(B) require an intact T-lymphocyte population
(C) show dermal infiltrates of granulocytes
(D) are associated uniquely with small antigens
(E) do not require previous exposure to the antigen

77. An adult migrant farm worker in the San Joaquin Valley of California has been hospitalized for 2 weeks with progressing lassitude, fever of unknown origin, and skin nodules on the lower extremities. A biopsy of one of the deep dermal nodules shown in the photomicrograph below reveals the presence of

(A) Russell bodies
(B) malignant lymphoma
(C) coccidioides spherule
(D) lymphomatoid granulomatosis
(E) erythema nodosum

---

78. The abnormality most compatible with a diagnosis of von Gierke's disease is a deficiency of

(A) glucose-6-phosphatase
(B) branching enzyme
(C) glucose-6-phosphate dehydrogenase
(D) muscle phosphorylase
(E) lysosomal glucosidase

79. Unusual characteristics of mycobacteria, such as resistance to toxic agents, environmental viability, and unusual stain reactions, can be attributed to their

(A) acid fastness
(B) aerobic requirements
(C) high lipid content
(D) peptidoglycan content
(E) plasma membrane

80. Togaviruses cause all the following disorders EXCEPT

(A) epidemic keratoconjunctivitis
(B) dengue
(C) eastern encephalitis
(D) yellow fever
(E) St. Louis encephalitis

81. All the following statements about *Mycobacterium tuberculosis* are true EXCEPT

(A) it has a long doubling time
(B) its cell wall contains large amounts of lipid
(C) it frequently infects silica miners
(D) it is prone to drug-resistant mutation
(E) it is a facultative anaerobe

82. Which of the following drugs may cause bronchospasm?

(A) Bleomycin
(B) Methotrexate
(C) Nitrofurantoin
(D) Aspirin
(E) Amiodarone

83. All the following diseases are associated with herpesviruses EXCEPT

(A) shingles
(B) chickenpox (varicella)
(C) influenza
(D) cytomegalic inclusion disease
(E) mononucleosis

84. The organism *Mycoplasma pneumoniae* exhibits all the following characteristics EXCEPT which one?

(A) It is enclosed by a membrane but lacks cell walls
(B) It causes 50 percent of pneumonias in college students
(C) It is often accompanied by the presence of cold agglutinins in serum
(D) It is beyond resolution of light microscopy
(E) It causes granuloma formation

85. A woman taking oral contraceptives during the reproductive years increases, even if only minimally, her risk of developing all the following EXCEPT

(A) pulmonary infarction
(B) myocardial infarction
(C) vaginal adenosis
(D) venous thrombus
(E) liver cell adenoma

86. Alcohol may be the most significant cause of public health problems in the United States. All the following entities are correlated with alcohol abuse EXCEPT

(A) subdural hematoma
(B) esophageal carcinoma
(C) elevated creatine phosphokinase
(D) primary biliary cirrhosis
(E) portal vein thrombosis

87. All the following statements about *Listeria monocytogenes* are true EXCEPT that it

(A) causes neonatal and adult men-
    ingitis
(B) causes food-borne outbreaks
(C) causes frequent epithelioid gran-
    ulomas
(D) is an opportunistic agent in the
    immunosuppressed or pregnant
(E) is a gram-positive intracellular
    bacillus

88. Current knowledge concerning AIDS (acquired immunodeficiency syndrome) includes all the following EXCEPT

(A) the causative agent is HIV
(B) the causative agent belongs to
    the retrovirus group
(C) T lymphocytes of the helper/in-
    ducer subset are infected
(D) cytotoxic/suppressor T cells are
    markedly increased
(E) lymphoid interstitial pneumoni-
    tis is seen in pediatric AIDS

---

89. The photomicrograph below shows cells found in a specimen of sputum sent for cytologic examination; no history except age (55) and sex (male) was supplied. True statements about the diagnosed condition include all the following EXCEPT

(A) location is most often hilar or central
(B) the abnormal cells suggest a leukemic process
(C) the cells are usually positive for neuroendocrine markers
(D) a paraneoplastic syndrome such as hyponatremia may be present
(E) origin is from argentaffin cells of the bronchial epithelium

90. A significant deficiency in vitamin D might be expected to lead to

(A) hyperostosis
(B) relative excess of osteoid tissue
(C) increased absorption of calcium
(D) decreased production of bone matrix
(E) adequate serum phosphorus

91. Infectious diseases associated with a granulomatous response include all the following EXCEPT

(A) tuberculosis
(B) coccidioidomycosis
(C) schistosomiasis
(D) sarcoidosis → *not-infection disease*
(E) cat-scratch disease

92. The photomicrograph below shows a labeling phenomenon of dark cytoplasmic granules within select cells. This staining technique has all the following characteristics EXCEPT

(A) it relies on neutral polysaccharides for a positive reaction
(B) it relies on antigen-antibody binding
(C) it may be used to identify proteins
(D) it may be used to identify tumor cell markers
(E) it may be used to identify viruses and other microorganisms

93. True statements about endometrial adenocarcinoma include all the following EXCEPT

(A) it is more common than invasive squamous cervical cancer
(B) it causes fewer deaths than invasive cervical cancer
(C) the peak incidence is at age 55 to 65 years
(D) the major symptom is pain
(E) abnormal glucose tolerance is a risk factor

94. Secondary gout may be seen in association with all the following EXCEPT

(A) polycythemia
(B) psoriasis
(C) hemolytic anemias
(D) myeloproliferative diseases
(E) chondrocalcinosis

95. Atherosclerosis, the most prevalent form of arterial disease in humans, is first manifested by an innocuous fatty streaking of the intima and is characterized by all the following EXCEPT

(A) onset in mid-life
(B) formation of essential lesions in the intima
(C) disintegration of the internal elastic lamina in advanced lesions
(D) relatively numerous lesions in larger arteries and fewer in smaller arteries
(E) plaque formations that cause little reduction in the luminal size of large arteries

96. Characteristics of granular cell tumors commonly include all the following EXCEPT

(A) location in the tongue
(B) PAS-positive, diastase-resistant granules
(C) association with pseudoepitheliomatous hyperplasia
(D) frequent malignant change
(E) origin from Schwann cell precursors

97. True statements regarding hemochromatosis include all the following EXCEPT

(A) it characteristically causes a micronodular pigment cirrhosis
(B) it is complicated by carcinoma of the liver in 15 to 30 percent of cases with cirrhosis
(C) it causes diabetes with severity unrelated to the degree of pancreatic iron deposition
(D) it can be diagnosed by liver biopsy showing raised amounts of hemosiderin
(E) it is associated with skin pigmentation due entirely to deposition of hemosiderin

98. As a result of active world travel, parasitic infestations are far from being considered exotic diseases in the United States today. A pulmonary phase is part of the development of all the following helminths EXCEPT

(A) *Necator americanus*
(B) *Strongyloides stercoralis*
(C) *Ascaris lumbricoides*
(D) *Wuchereria bancrofti*
(E) *Toxocara*

99. All the following functions can be attributed to the cell depicted in the electron photomicrograph below EXCEPT

(A) production of thromboplastin
(B) production of interleukin I
(C) synthesis of factor VIII-vWF
(D) production of collagenase
(E) production of components of complement

100. Taking patient discomfort and expense into account, bone marrow aspiration and trephine examination are indicated to document all the following EXCEPT

(A) metastatic carcinoma
(B) iron deficiency anemia
(C) sideroblastic anemia
(D) osteomalacia
(E) the amount of bone in the sample

101. An increased incidence of neoplasia has been observed in all the following EXCEPT

(A) primary (genetic) immunodeficient states
(B) immunosuppressed recipients of transplants
(C) acquired immunodeficiency syndrome (AIDS)
(D) therapy with radiation and radiomimetic drugs
(E) sarcoidosis

102. Organisms that can cause summertime infections around coastal areas of the United States and are characterized microscopically by a curved bacillus include

(A) *Mycobacterium avium*
(B) *Mycobacterium bovis*
(C) *Mycobacterium marinum*
(D) *Vibrio cholerae*
(E) *Mycobacterium kansasii*

103. Leukotrienes differ from prostaglandins in the mediation of inflammation by more potent actions in all the following EXCEPT

(A) chemotaxis
(B) vasoconstriction
(C) bronchoconstriction
(D) edema formation
(E) vascular permeability

104. Clinical risk factors for development of carcinoma of the female breast include all the following EXCEPT

(A) early menopause
(B) nulliparity
(C) history of endometrial cancer
(D) early menarche
(E) obesity

Questions 105–107

For each of the disorders listed, choose the most appropriate feature.

(A) Mental retardation and self-mutilation
(B) Deficiency of α-galactosidase A
(C) Second most common cause of genetic mental retardation
(D) Situs inversus
(E) Deficiency of hexosaminidase A

105. Fabry's disease

106. Tay-Sachs disease

107. Fragile X syndrome

Questions 108–111

Match each vitamin deficiency with the disorder with which it is most likely to be associated.

(A) Microcytic anemia
(B) Perifollicular petechiae
(C) Wernicke-Korsakoff syndrome
(D) Macrocytic anemia
(E) Night blindness

108. Pyridoxine deficiency

109. Ascorbic acid deficiency

110. Folate deficiency

111. Thiamine deficiency

Questions 112–115

Match the following characteristics and diseases.

(A) Tick-borne disease
(B) Granulomatous inflammation
(C) Meningitis
(D) Mosquito-borne disease
(E) Endotoxins in cell walls

112. Histoplasmosis

113. Cryptococcosis

114. Rocky Mountain spotted fever

115. Yellow fever

Questions 116–119

For each disease causative of blindness, select the characteristic with which it is most likely to be associated.

(A) Silver-wire arterioles
(B) Variable modes of inheritance
(C) Microaneurysms
(D) Bitot's spots
(E) Pannus formation

116. Diabetic retinopathy

117. Keratomalacia

118. Trachoma

119. Retinitis pigmentosa

Questions 120–123

Match each disorder or description with the immunoglobulin with which it is most likely to be associated.

(A) IgA
(B) IgD
(C) IgE
(D) IgM
(E) IgG

120. Anaphylaxis

121. The major circulating immunoglobulin

122. Berger's disease

123. Waldenström's macroglobulinemia

General Pathology

Answers

1. The answer is A. (*Robbins, 4/e. pp 31–33.*) In uterine growth during pregnancy, both cell proliferation involving the endometrial glands and muscle enlargement of the uterine wall occur. These processes offer models of both hyperplasia and hypertrophy. When both are present, DNA synthesis is markedly accelerated. Hyperplasia is an increase in the number of cells, whereas hypertrophy is an increase in cell size, as in cardiac muscle hypertrophy in response to volume overload or peripheral vascular hypertension. Breast tissue enlargement resulting from hormonal influences is due solely to an increase in cell numbers.

2. The answer is C. (*Robbins, 4/e. pp 78–80, 138–139.*) Type I collagen is found in skin, tendon, bone, dentin, and fascia; type II collagen is found only in cartilage; type III collagen (reticulin) appears in skin, blood vessels, uterus, and embryonic dermis. Type IV collagen, a component of basement laminae of epithelial and endothelial cells, does not have the typical 67-nm banding of types I, II, and III. Synthesis of collagen includes lysine oxidation, resulting in alpha-chain cross-linkages with structural stability of collagen. Decreased formation of cross-linkages in collagen and elastin occurs in Marfan's syndrome, an autosomal dominant disorder of connective tissues, with skeletal abnormalities including arachnodactyly, lens subluxation, and cystic medionecrosis of aorta with aneurysm and sometimes rupture.

3. The answer is B. (*Robbins, 4/e. pp 4–9.*) Injury to the cell membrane, the loss of cell ATP, and the influx of Ca^{2+} into the mitochondria are thought to be the most critical of multiple cellular events after experimental ischemia in animals. A major detriment following reduction of cell oxygen tension is the cessation or reduction in ATP because of falling oxidative phosphorylation; this occurs early in hypoxia. While increasing anaerobic glycolysis subsequently occurs, the pivotal step is loss of the energy-producing ATP, which leads to cell Na^+ accumulation, K^+ efflux, and Ca^{2+} influx, by reduced effectiveness of the active transport Na^+ pump. Cells greatly enlarge as a consequence of isoosmotic water accumulation. These changes are still reversible if oxygen tension is restored. Continuing hypoxia results in mitochondrial damage (vacuole formation), which is irreversible. Cell death will occur when lysosomes break down and release proteases, RNA and DNAases, and cathepsins. Central nervous system cells are most susceptible to ischemia (5 min or less), while liver and kidney cells survive up to 2 h with epidermal cells tolerating several hours of hypoxia.

4.   The answer is E. *(Robbins, 4/e. pp 45–46.)* Leukocyte function antigen 1 (LFA-1) is one of the group of adhesive molecules on leukocytes. Other members of this group, all glycoproteins and all having identical β chains, are MO-1 and P-150. A genetic deficiency of the β-chain adhesive proteins on leukocytes (leukocyte adhesion deficiency) results in impaired leukocyte adhesion and recurrent bacterial infections. Endothelial leukocyte adhesion molecule (ELAM-1) is one of the adhesive surface proteins on endothelial cells. Complement fragments (C5a) and leukotriene B4 are mediators that stimulate an increase in adhesive molecules on *leukocytes*. Conversely, interleukin 1 (IL-1) stimulates leukocytic adhesion by action on adhesive surface proteins on *endothelial* cells. Tumor necrosis factor (TNF) stimulates adhesive molecules on *both* leukocytes and endothelial cells.

5.   The answer is C. *(Robbins, 4/e. pp 58–60, 70–71, 168–169, 183.)* Two of the major systemic effects of inflammation (acute-phase reactions) are fever and leukocytosis. Both of these reactions are largely under the control of the cytokines IL-1 or α-TNF (cachectin) or both. These two cytokines have many similar functions, including induction of fever, release of ACTH, leukocytosis, and other systemic acute-phase responses. IL-1 initiates fever by inducing synthesis of prostaglandin E_2 (PGE_2) in the anterior hypothalamus, followed by transmission via the posterior hypothalamus, vasomotor center, and sympathetic nerves to cause skin vasoconstriction. Leukocytosis occurs initially because of rapid release of cells from the postmitotic reserve pool of the bone marrow, which is caused by IL-1 and α-TNF and associated with a "shift to the left" of immature cells. β-TNF, another cytokine, has no major role in acute-phase reactions. It takes part in T-cell cytotoxicity and its release may injure cell membranes directly in T-cell–mediated lysis.

6.   The answer is B. *(Robbins, 4/e. pp 51–52.)* The enzymatic defect that exists in chronic granulomatous disease of childhood does not impair chemotaxis or the cell's ability to engulf bacteria but rather involves a failure to produce hydrogen peroxide after engulfment. Chemotactic defects resulting in inhibition of the capacity of leukocytes to infiltrate an area of infection or injury may be due to intracellular defects, as found in Chédiak-Higashi syndrome, in other genetic defects, and in diabetes mellitus. Chronic renal failure and cirrhosis may be associated with factors in the circulation that impair chemotaxis. Whether newborn infants are full-term or immature, neonatal leukocytes have a temporary chemotactic defect that is corrected with increasing age.

7.   The answer is C. *(Takahashi, 2/e. pp 305–306.)* In the cluster of cells shown, marked variation in cell size, nuclear hyperchromatism, and prominent nuclear membranes can be seen and are diagnostic characteristics of malignancy. The tendency of cells to cluster and overlap, the prominent nucleoli, and the vacuolated cytoplasm are signs that strongly support a diagnosis of adenocarcinoma rather than oat cell carcinoma.

8.   The answer is C. *(Robbins, 4/e. pp 29–30, 51–52.)* Cytoskeletal filament proteins compose the framework of cells involved in cell functions, such as pinocytosis, structural stability, contractility, organelle movement, and cell motility. The cytoskeleton is seen ultrastructurally as microtubules (25 nm diameter) of tubulin protein; intermediate filaments (8 to 10 nm) of keratins, desmin, vimentin, glial and neurofilaments; thin filaments of actin (6 to 8 nm); and thick filaments (15 nm) of myosin. Every cell has tubulin and actin, while most have some myosin. Epithelial cells have any of the many types of cytokeratins, with a few having the mesenchymal filament vimentin. Muscle cells and fibroblasts have desmin. Glial cells and neurons contain glial and neurofilament protein, respectively. Phagocytosis is impaired in the Chédiak-Higashi syndrome because of a defect in the polymerization of microtubules. Alcoholic "hyaline" (Mallory's bodies) in alcoholic liver disease appears to be composed of prekeratins. Red cells have a membrane skeleton made up of spectrin, ankyrin, actin, and protein 4.1. In hereditary spherocytosis a genetic defect is responsible for abnormal spectrin that is unable to bind protein 4.1 required for the stability of the red cell membrane.

9.   The answer is D. *(Robbins, 4/e. pp 114–119.)* Septic shock is caused by the gram-negative, endotoxin-producing aerobic rods mentioned in the question. It results from pooling of blood in the peripheral circulation. A common cause of sepsis in burn wounds is *Pseudomonas aeruginosa*. The major target in severe shock is the kidneys, which suffer acute ischemic tubular necrosis, affecting proximal and distal nephrons in septic shock. Gram-negative endotoxic shock has a 70 percent mortality.

10. The answer is D. *(Anderson, 9/e. pp 2154–2156. Henry, 18/e. pp 456–457.)* In a patient who is suspected of having meningitis, microscopic examination of cerebrospinal fluid is of immediate importance. In the photomicrograph shown, all the cells are polymorphonuclear leukocytes and bacteria are visible in the cytoplasm. Neutrophils may be present in viral or tuberculous meningitis, but lymphocytes are more common. Demonstration of bacteria by Gram stain of the cerebrospinal fluid is the most valuable aid in establishing a diagnosis of early bacterial meningitis and is possible in more than 90 percent of cases.

11. The answer is E. *(Robbins, 4/e. pp 52–60.)* Lysosomes contain many substances involved in inflammation including alkaline and acid phosphatase, collagenases, lysozymes, lactoferrin, myeloperoxidase, cationic proteins, and acid proteases. Of these, the neutral proteases (elastase, collagenase, cathepsin G) function in stages of inflammatory confinement and wound healing by degrading tissue matrix like collagen, fibrin, cartilage, elastin, and basement membranes. The other mediators cascade as follows: complement cascade starts classically by an antigen-antibody complex or alternately by non-immunologic stimuli. C5a leads to chemotaxis while the complement complex C5b-9 leads to cell lysis. The kinins are activated by Hageman factor (XIIA), via prekallikrein, into bradykinin. The fibrinopeptides of the clotting system can also be activated by Hageman factor or by extrinsic tissue thromboplastin to result in a polymerized fibrin clot. The important cascades of arachidonic acid metabolites (cyclooxygenase, lipoxygenase), leading to functioning vasodilators (prostaglandins) and membrane permeability factors (leukotrienes), are the most complex of all, beginning with the actions of phospholipase.

12. The answer is D. *(Robbins, 4/e. pp 818–821.)* Carcinoma of the oral cavity accounts for approximately 5 percent of all human malignancies. More than 90 percent are squamous cell type and precursor lesions include leukoplakia and erythroplasia (dysplastic leukoplakia) with transformation rates of approximately 15 and 50 percent, respectively. It is more common in males. Smoking, tobacco chewing, chronic irritation, heat exposure, and irradiation are all thought to contribute to carcinogenesis. The lower lip is the most common site followed by the floor of the mouth, anterior tongue, palate, and posterior tongue. Prognosis varies according to site but is best for lesions of the lip and worst for lesions in the floor of the mouth.

13. The answer is D. *(Anderson, 9/e. pp 438–439.)* *Giardia lamblia*, a flagellate protozoan, is the most common cause of outbreaks of waterborne diarrheal disease in the U.S. and is seen frequently in Rocky Mountain areas. Ingestion of cysts from contaminated water results in trophozoites in duodenum and jejunum. Identification of the trophozoite stage is done by duodenal aspiration or small-bowel biopsy and of the cyst stage (intermittent) by examination of stool. The trophozoite may appear as a pear-shaped, binucleate organism ("two eyes"). Giardiasis may cause malabsorption but is often asymptomatic. Duodenal aspiration, immunofluorescence, and ELISA testing for *Giardia* antigens are diagnostic and therapy with metronidazole or quinacrine is effective. Lymph nodes often contain numerous parasites in trypanosomiasis and leishmaniasis. *Triatoma* is the vector of Chagas' disease (American trypanosomiasis). *Trichomonas vaginalis* is identified in cervicovaginal smears.

14. The answer is C. *(Robbins, 4/e. pp 1374–1375.)* Liposarcomas are the most common soft tissue sarcoma of adults, arise deeply in thigh or retroperitoneum, and are liable to metastasize by embolization in blood vessels (nonmyxoid types). Histology is varied: well-differentiated, myxoid, round cell, or pleomorphic—depending on tumor type. Myxoid liposarcoma is the most common variant. The pleomorphic type is undifferentiated and easily confused with other poorly differentiated mesenchymal sarcomas. The clinical picture is also varied. Well-differentiated and myxoid types are locally invasive and recurrent, if they are not completely excised, but they are rarely metastatic. Round-cell and pleomorphic types are often aggressive with widespread metastases, local recurrence, and poor 5-year survival.

15. The answer is D. *(Robbins, 4/e. pp 61–63.)* There is evidence that most, if not all, macrophages originate from a committed bone marrow stem cell, which differentiates into a monoblast and then a promonocyte, which in turn matures into a monocyte in the circulating peripheral blood. When called upon, the circulating monocyte can enter into an organ or tissue bed as a tissue macrophage (previously called a *histiocyte*). Examples of tissue macrophages are Kupffer cells (liver), alveolar macrophages (lung), osteoclasts (bone), Langerhans cells (skin), microglial cells (central nervous system), and possibly the dendritic immunocytes of the dermis, spleen, and lymph nodes. The entire system, including the peripheral blood monocytes, constitutes the mononuclear phagocyte system.

16. The answer is B. *(Anderson, 9/e. p 1474.)* The lymph-node section shown in the photomicrograph contains metastatic carcinoma cells and was probably excised from a patient who has carcinoma. The tumor cells are clustered in small nests within the node and are separated by stromal tissue. The cellular clustering is characteristic of carcinomas that have metastasized to lymph nodes.

17. The answer is A. *(Robbins, 4/e. pp 146–148.)* Sphingomyelin, a lipid composed of phosphocholine and a ceramide, characteristically is found in abnormally high concentrations throughout the body tissues of patients who have any one of the forms of Niemann-Pick disease. Division of this disease into five categories is generally accepted; type A, the acute neuronopathic form, is the one that has the highest incidence. The lack of sphingomyelinase in type A is the metabolic defect that prevents the hydrolytic cleavage of sphingomyelin, which then accumulates in the brain. Patients who have the type A form usually show hepatosplenomegaly at 6 months of age, progressively lose motor functions and mental capabilities, and die during the third year of life.

18. The answer is B. *(Robbins, 4/e. pp 745–747.)* The Hand-Schüller-Christian (HSC) disease is a complex of three syndromes affecting the reticuloendothelial system: Letterer-Siwe syndrome, Hand-Schüller-Christian syndrome, and eosinophilic granuloma. An unknown pathogenesis and an abnormal production of histiocytes are characteristics common to all three syndromes and provide the basis for the designation of HSC disease as *histiocytosis X* (the alternate term is *Langerhans cell granulomatosis,* since the cells have the Birbeck granules ultrastructurally, as do Langerhans cells).

19. The answer is A. *(Anderson, 9/e. p 874.)* The findings of small, firm testes, eunuchoidism, gynecomastia, and mental retardation constitute the classic manifestations of Klinefelter's syndrome, a type of hypogonadism. The seminiferous tubules may be sclerosed and hyalinized. Urinary levels of gonadotropin are usually elevated; the elevation is thought to result from the absence of controlling testicular hormones, not from pituitary dysfunction.

20. The answer is B. *(Robbins, 4/e. pp 127, 136.)* Mendel's laws deal with single-gene mutations that may be inherited or acquired de novo, with expression of the abnormality highly variable. In autosomal dominance inheritances, if a mutant gene is unexpressed, this is called *reduced penetrance* and it may vary by a percentage that reflects the degree of expression. *Variable expressivity* refers to expression of the trait in all who harbor the mutant gene, but with different expressions of the abnormality. *Nondisjunction* refers to a failure of disjoining of a homologous pair of chromosomes during meiosis (may result in aneuploidy). *Codominance* refers to the full expression of both alleles of a gene pair. *Genetic heterogeneity* applies to multiple-loci mutations (each in a different location, reflecting multiple different mutations), which can result in the same or similar expressed abnormality.

21. The answer is E. *(Robbins, 4/e. pp 1377–1378.)* Fibrosarcomas are most frequent in the retroperitoneum, followed by the superficial or deep tissues of the extremities. They form one of the less common tumors of soft tissue since many previously diagnosed as fibrosarcoma have been reclassified as malignant fibrous histiocytoma or aggressive fibromatosis (desmoid). Slowly growing, well-differentiated fibrosarcomas may be difficult to differentiate from "cellular fibromas." Hypoglycemia may be associated with fibrosarcoma.

22. The answer is C. *(Williams, 4/e. pp 980–982.)* Cytopenias occur in over 50 percent of patients with HIV infection either individually or as part of a pancytopenia. Suppression of hemopoiesis in the bone marrow as a result of mycobacterial, fungal, or protozoal infection; infiltration by lymphoma, leukemia, or Kaposi's sarcoma; and the effects of drugs (particularly zidovudine) may result in cytopenia. Anemia is seen in up to 90 percent of cases, usually in the pattern of anemia of chronic disease. Thrombocytopenia occurs in up to 60 percent of cases and is thought to be a result of peripheral destruction of platelets, possibly by an immune mechanism. Neutropenia is common and is often secondary to use of zidovudine. Severely neutropenic patients often show eosinophilia rather than eosinopenia. Lymphopenia and a reduced ratio of CD4 to CD8 lymphocytes are characteristic of HIV infection. Examination of the bone marrow in cytopenic patients shows a normocellular or hypercellular pattern in more than 90 percent of cases.

23. The answer is A. (*Robbins, 4/e. pp 51–52, 223.*) The classic form of chronic granulomatous disease usually afflicts boys and causes their death before they reach the age of 10 years. Key findings in chronic granulomatous disease include lymphadenitis, hepatosplenomegaly, eczematoid dermatitis, pulmonary infiltrates that are associated with hypergammaglobulinemia, and defective ability of neutrophils to kill bacteria. The last finding is thought to be caused by a delay in the release of neutrophilic lysosomal enzymes responsible for intracellular bactericidal action. Although defective neutrophilic bactericidal action also is associated with the Chédiak-Higashi syndrome, this syndrome is distinguished by photophobia and oculocutaneous albinism. Thrombocytopenia is a feature of Wiskott-Aldrich syndrome.

24. The answer is C. (*Robbins, 4/e. pp 29, 945–946.*) Hyaline inclusions, as shown in the illustration, may appear in liver cells injured by chronic alcoholism and have been shown by ultrastructure studies to result from the close packing of fibrils. The appearance of these inclusions is not a morphologic expression of cell injury. Alcoholic hyaline inclusions (Mallory's bodies) are nonspecific and occur in Wilson's disease, Indian childhood cirrhosis, bypass operations for morbid obesity, and alcoholic hepatitis. They react with antibodies to cytokeratins, which suggests they are related to the intermediate filament keratin.

25. The answer is D. (*Robbins, 4/e. pp 177, 224–226, 296–297, 955–956.*) Newly discovered membrane surface antigens on the surfaces of neoplastic cells have stimulated interest and research. These tumor-associated antigens are largely glycoproteins (proteoglycans, chondroitins, heparin) that are at least anchored in the bilipid cell membrane with polypeptide chains emerging "into space" on the surface. Monoclonal antibodies can be raised against certain epitopes on the external portions of these surface antigens. Also the host may mount specific immunoglobulins against these sites. These antigens are membrane-associated, induce transplantation immunity, and are distinct from histocompatibility antigens; they are called *tumor-specific transplantation antigens (TSTAs)* or *tumor-associated rejection antigens (TARAs)*. TSTAs are found on tumor cells that were transformed by viral oncogenes. TSTAs resemble differentiation antigens in normal cells of some animal strains. Most TSTAs are related to carcinogens or oncogenes and are usually absent in spontaneous tumors. ADCC is antibody-dependent cell-mediated cytotoxicity; A1AT is alpha-1-antitrypsin. HIV is the designation of the AIDS retrovirus, while ARC is the AIDS-related complex.

26. The answer is E. (*Robbins, 4/e. p 259.*) Generally tumor cells, by virtue of their transformation, exhibit ultrastructural alterations as visualized by electron microscopy as well as physiologic changes. Membrane projections (microvilli, filopodia, pseudopodia) may become blunted, or lost altogether. Neoplastic transformation may be associated with formation of projections in some cells, but the loss of attenuation of surface projections is more characteristic of neoplastic cells. Cytoskeletal microfilaments and tubules become disorganized, while intermediate filaments (keratins, desmin, vimentin) may increase. In addition to formation of membrane-associated glycoproteins (tumor antigens), there is increased "shedding" and loss of surface antigens. Fibronectin, for instance, is lost from tumor cell surfaces and may be measured in the patient's plasma as cold-insoluble globulin. Surface glycolipids (many are receptor sites) are diminished or lost in some neoplastic cells, theoretically enabling tumor cells to escape the growth inhibitory effects of chalones. Plant lectins can agglutinate cells because their property of divalency cross-links sugars on neighboring cells. This lectin agglutinability is increased in many malignant cells. Fundamental to the biologic behavior of neoplastic cells is the increased demand for cell nutrients, which is aided by an observed increase in membrane transport in neoplastic cells.

27. The answer is A. (*Anderson, 9/e. p 492. Robbins, 4/e. pp 165–167.*) With the advent of monoclonal antibodies derived from hybridomas, it is now possible to identify cells of certain specificity. These antibodies recognize epitopes of antigens found on the cell surfaces that have been used to induce immunity within the mouse. Using an immunoperoxidase technique, the OKT (Leu series) identifies T cells. In addition specific markers will identify subsets of T cells. For example, all peripheral blood T cells react with OKT1, OKT3, and OKT11 cluster designations CD5, CD3, and CD2; OKT4 (Leu-3) reacts with mature T cells; OKT4 or CD4 identifies helper T cells; and OKT8 (CD8) reacts with suppressor cells. The normal T helper/suppressor ratio in humans is about 2. These antibodies do not label cells other than those in the T-lymphocyte system. T cells as a group function in immune regulation and act in concert with B lymphocytes and macrophages. T helper cells aid the cellular immune response in reaction to antigens, while T suppressor cells help in turning the immune response off. EAC rosette cells refer to B lymphocytes that have surface receptors (C3b) that bind to sheep erythrocytes coated with IgM antibody and complement. B lymphocytes also express surface immunoglobulin.

28. The answer is B. *(Robbins, 4/e. pp 50–51, 167–168, 297, 299.)* The enzyme myeloperoxidase is found in high concentration in neutrophilic granulocytes and exerts strong antibacterial effects by combining with chloride and hydrogen peroxide. Natural killer (NK) cells are able to lyse certain tumor cells, virus-infected cells, fungi, and some normal cells without prior sensitization. It is now believed that most so-called killer (K) cells are really NK cells, and K cells are now known as *cytotoxic T cells*. NK cells lyse target cells in two ways: through direct cytotoxicity by means of their NK receptors, and through antibody-dependent cytotoxicity (ADCC) by their Fc receptors for IgG. NK cells are sometimes called *large granular lymphocytes* (larger than small lymphocytes); their granules contain lytic substances but not myeloperoxidase. NK cells share some surface antigens with T cells and macrophages but are considered distinct from these. Monoclonal antibodies reacting with NK cells include CD16. Following activation and increase in numbers by culture with IL-2, NK cells can kill many tumor cells, and these lymphokine-activated killer (LAK) cells are being evaluated in the immunotherapy of some cancers—leukemia, melanoma, renal cell carcinoma—currently treated with IL-2 and interferons.

29. The answer is D. *(Robbins, 4/e. pp 173–183.)* The type of reaction in the question is a type 2 hypersensitivity reaction that is mediated by antibodies reacting against antigens present on the surface of cells, in this case blood group antigens or irregular antigens present on the donor's red blood cells. Type 2 hypersensitivity reactions result from attachment of antibodies to changed cell surface antigens or to normal cell surface antigens. Complement-mediated cytotoxicity occurs when IgM or IgG binds to a cell surface antigen with complement activation and consequent cell membrane damage or lysis. Blood transfusion reactions and autoimmune hemolytic anemia are examples of this form. Systemic anaphylaxis is a type 1 hypersensitivity reaction in which mast cells or basophils that are bound to IgE antibodies are reexposed to an allergen, which leads to a release of vasoactive amines that causes edema and broncho- and vasoconstriction. Sudden death can occur. Systemic immune complex reactions are found in type 3 reactions and are due to circulating antibodies that form complexes upon reexposure to an antigen, such as foreign serum, which then activates complement followed by chemotaxis and aggregation of neutrophils leading to release of lysosomal enzymes and eventual necrosis of tissue and cells. Serum sickness and Arthus' reactions are examples of this. Delayed-type hypersensitivity is type 4 and is due to previously sensitized T lymphocytes, which release lymphokines upon reexposure to the antigen. This takes time—perhaps up to several days following exposure. The tuberculin reaction is the best known example of this. T cell–mediated cytotoxicity leads to lysis of cells by cytotoxic T cells in response to tumor cells, allogenic tissue, and virus-infected cells. These cells have CD8 antigens on their surfaces.

30. The answer is C. *(Anderson, 9/e. pp 209–213.)* Heavy metal poisoning may occur via the respiratory route owing to contaminated inhalant and vapors. Such poisoning is usually industrially related, as with mercury (calomel workers), arsenic (pesticides), and lead (batteries and paints). Cadmium has been implicated in producing not only an acute form of pneumonia, but, with chronic exposure to small concentrations of cadmium vapors, diffuse interstitial pulmonary fibrosis and an increased incidence of emphysema as well. The "honeycomb" radiologic pattern is indicative of an interstitial fibrotic process and may be the result of repeated pneumonitis and bronchitis. Cadmium can also be found in tobacco smoke. Cobalt poisoning leads to myocardiopathy, mercury poisoning leads to renal tubular damage, and lead poisoning leads to liver necrosis and cerebral edema. Arsenic poisoning, in addition to carrying an increased risk of lung and skin cancer, may produce death caused by inhibition of respiratory enzymes and cardiac subendocardial hemorrhages complicated by gastroenteritis with shock.

31. The answer is C. *(Anderson, 9/e. pp 531–532.)* An allograft is also called a *homograft* and refers to a graft between members of the same species. An autograft is a tissue graft taken from one site and placed in a different site in the same individual. Isografts are grafts between individuals from an inbred strain of animals. A graft between individuals of two different species is a xenograft, or heterograft.

32. The answer is C. *(Robbins, 4/e. pp 209–209.)* Fifteen to twenty percent of cases of polymyositis are associated with underlying visceral malignancies of virtually any organ. Although the cause of this association remains unknown, it has been postulated that some cancers either produce substances that are toxic to skeletal muscle or contain antigens that are cross-reactive with skeletal muscle.

33. The answer is D. *(Robbins, 4/e. pp 194–194, 205.)* Diagnostic specificity is defined as the probability of a negative diagnostic test result in the absence of the disease the test is designed to detect, or, simply, the ability of a screening test to correctly identify a person who is free of the specific disease. Two clinically useful tests specific for systemic lupus erythematosus (SLE) are the detection of antibodies to double-stranded DNA (anti-ds DNA) and to the nonhistone Smith (Sm) antigen, since these antibodies are rare in other autoimmune diseases. Positive testing for antinuclear antibody (ANA) occurs in virtually all patients with SLE (marked diagnostic sensitivity), but the test is *not specific* since positive results are frequent in other autoimmune diseases. In diffuse systemic sclerosis, positive antibodies to nucleolar RNA and Scl-70 antibody to nonhistone nuclear protein are specific. In the CREST syndrome of systemic sclerosis, an anticentromere antibody is specific. The best information from laboratory tests comes from their positive and negative predictive values (PVs) relating the results (+ or −) to prevalence of the disease in the population being studied.

34. The answer is B. *(Robbins, 4/e. pp 196–201.)* Renal failure is the most common cause of death in SLE. Most cases show some renal abnormality (mild or marked) by immunofluorescence and by light and electron microscopy. Diffuse proliferative glomerulonephritis (GN) occurs in about 50 percent of cases and is the most common and most serious renal lesion. Subendothelial location of immune complex deposits is particularly characteristic of SLE. Membranous GN occurs in only 10 percent of cases and has a better prognosis, but may progress. Polyclonal B-cell activation occurs with increased production of autoantibodies and hypergammaglobulinemia. This B-cell activation may follow genetic B-cell abnormalities or loss of T-suppressor cell influence. Most of the tissue lesions are mediated by the immune complex (type III hypersensitivity). Nonerosive arthritis occurs in about 90 percent of cases and often involves small peripheral joints. Lack of deformity and of synovial proliferation distinguish arthritis of SLE from rheumatoid arthritis.

35. The answer is C. *(Robbins, 4/e. pp 202–204.)* Sjögren's syndrome is characterized by dryness of the mouth (xerostomia) and eyes (keratoconjunctivitis sicca). Secondary Sjögren's syndrome is associated with rheumatoid arthritis (RA), or SLE, or systemic sclerosis. The primary form shows increased frequency of HLA-DR3, while association with RA shows a positive correlation with HLA-DR4. Anti-SSB antibodies are fairly specific, anti-SSA less so, and both may occur in SLE; rheumatoid factor is often present. Glomerular lesions are very rare but a mild tubulointerstitial nephritis is quite common and may result in renal tubular acidosis. In addition to the usual dense, lymphoplasmacytic infiltrate of salivary glands, the lymph nodes may show a "pseudolymphomatous" appearance. True B-cell lymphomas have developed with increased frequency in Sjögren's syndrome (relative risk of 44).

36. The answer is E. *(Robbins, 4/e. pp 183–188.)* Histocompatible antigens (HLA) are responsible for rejection of transplanted organs in humans. Organ rejection requires both humoral and cell-mediated immunologic reactions involving T cells both from the donated organ and the patient's own CD4 T helper cells and CD8 cytotoxic T cells. Hyperacute rejection occurs within minutes after transplantation and consists of neutrophils within the glomerulus and peritubular capillaries. Acute rejection occurs within days after transplantation and is marked by vasculitis and interstitial lymphocytic infiltration. Subacute rejection vasculitis occurs during the first few months after transplantation and is characterized by the proliferation of fibroblasts and macrophages in the tunica intima of arteries. In chronic rejection tubular atrophy, mononuclear interstitial infiltration, and vascular changes are encountered, with the vascular changes being characteristic and probably reflecting an end stage of arteritis. The vascular obliteration leads to interstitial fibrosis and tubular atrophy with loss of renal function. However, the histologic picture is complicated by secondary ischemic damage, and it may be difficult to discern inflammation, fibrosis, and vascular changes as cause or effect.

37. The answer is C. *(Robbins, 4/e. pp 366–367, 1355.)* A localized skin rash in the summertime followed within a period of weeks by arthritis, especially involving less than three joints, should arouse suspicion of Lyme disease. This disorder was first described in the mid-1970s in Connecticut when small clusters of cases of children suffering from an illness resembling juvenile rheumatoid arthritis were first noted. The disease has now been shown to be caused by a spirochete, *Borrelia burgdorferi,* through the bite of a tick belonging to the genus *Ixodes*. The spirochete-infested ticks reside in forested areas where there are deer and small rodents. The deer act as a wintering-over reservoir for the ticks. In the spring the tick larval stage emerges and evolves into a nymph, which is infective for humans if they are bitten. Adult ticks are also capable of transmitting the spirochete as well during questing. The bite is followed by a rash called *erythema chronicum migrans,* which may resolve spontaneously. However, many patients have a transient phase of spirochetemia, which may allow the spread of the spirochete to the meninges, heart, and synovial tissue. Originally thought to be confined to New England, Lyme disease has now been shown to be present in Europe and Australia as well. The spirochetes are sensitive to penicillin, erythromycin, and tetracycline. Reiter's disease does not present with a spreading rash, and a Baker's cyst produces swelling in the popliteal fossa behind the knee rather than joint effusions anteriorly.

38. The answer is C. *(Robbins, 4/e. p 1333.)* Hypertrophic osteoarthropathy is a syndrome consisting of periosteal new bone formation with, or without, digital clubbing and joint effusion. It is seen usually in an adult who complains of aching bone pain, especially in distal extremities. While it is most common in association with lung carcinoma (up to 10 percent of cases), it also occurs with pleural mesothelioma, chronic lung disease such as bronchiectasis or lung abscess, infective endocarditis, and, less commonly, with cirrhosis or inflammatory bowel disease (ulcerative colitis). It may occur with congenital heart, lung, or liver disease in children and in familial and idiopathic forms. Radiographs show periosteal thickening with new bone formation on diaphyseal ends of long bones. Treatment is that of the associated disorder, the arthropathy being reversible with surgical resection or medical correction of the underlying disease.

39. The answer is C. (*Anderson, 9/e. pp 1255–1256.*) Antibodies to mitochondria are not present in the serum of patients who have acute viral hepatitis when immunofluorescent techniques are used. Serum antibodies to mitochondria are present, however, in 87 percent of patients who have primary biliary cirrhosis, 69 percent of patients who have chlorpromazine-induced jaundice, 66 percent of patients who have chronic active hepatitis, and 18 percent of patients who have systemic lupus erythematosus. Immunofluorescent detection techniques for antibodies to mitochondria are not specific for one particular disease, but, when evaluated in conjunction with tests for antinuclear antibodies and antibodies to smooth muscle, they can be helpful in differential diagnosis.

40. The answer is D. (*Robbins, 4/e. pp 133–135.*) The Barr body represents a sex chromatin clump attached to the nuclear membrane that originates from an entire X chromosome and can easily be seen by using light microscopy to examine scrapings of the epithelium of the inside buccal mucosa. According to the formula $M = n - 1$, the total number of X chromatin masses equals the number of cellular X chromatin masses seen in the nucleus minus 1. Hence, normal males are $0 = 1 - 1$ (no Barr body), and normal females are $1 = 2 - 1$ (one Barr body). In classic Turner's syndrome (XO), the expected buccal smear would be $0 = 1 - 1$ (no Barr bodies seen), as in a normal male. Karyotyping is necessary when the Barr body screening test is ambiguous or inconclusive. In a young woman of short stature and average intelligence who has never menstruated, there is a strong indication that one of the forms of Turner's syndrome exists, and the presence of one Barr body indicates that the patient has XX in some percentage of cells. About 10 percent of all Turner's syndrome patients show a mosaic pattern, with some cells having XO/XX or XO/XXX patterns. In this example, the patient is likely to be XO/XX by the formula $1 = 2 - 1$. In Turner's mosaics, the likelihood of developing a seminoma or gonadoblastoma is higher than expected, and gonadectomy may be indicated.

41. The answer is A. *(Henry, 18/e. pp 224–225.)* C-reactive protein (CRP) elevations, as well as elevations in the erythrocyte sedimentation rate, are nonspecific markers of inflammatory conditions. The CRP rises faster and returns to normal earlier than the erythrocyte sedimentation rate in most inflammatory diseases. Most bacterial infections, rheumatoid arthritis, rheumatic fever, and diseases leading to necrosis and tissue damage will elevate the CRP. CRP elevations do not occur in most viral illnesses.

42. The answer is C. *(Robbins, 4/e. p 369.)* Although the rapid plasma reagin (RPR), Kolmer, and Venereal Disease Research Laboratory (VDRL) tests are rapid and easily performed tests that can help confirm a diagnosis of active syphilis, they are associated with false positive reactions because of their low specificity for antibodies against treponemal or cardiolipin antigens. Therefore, RPR, Kolmer, and VDRL tests usually are used for screening programs. The *Treponema pallidum* immobilization (TPI) and the fluorescent treponemal antibody-absorption (FTA-ABS) tests have greater specificity for treponemal antigen but are technically more difficult to perform. The FTA-ABS test is generally the most sensitive and most specific procedure for diagnosis of syphilis.

43. The answer is E. *(Robbins, 4/e. pp 380–382.)* Lepromatous and tuberculoid leprosy, the major forms, are caused by *Mycobacterium leprae* and nerve involvement is most typical of the lepromatous form. Numerous bacilli in packets occupy histiocytes or lepra cells in the lesions of lepromatous leprosy. Polyclonal hypergammaglobulinemia often occurs in lepromatous leprosy, in which patients do not have the adequate cellular immune response of the tuberculoid form. Large amounts of anti-lepra antibody occur in the lepromatous form with frequent formation of antigen-antibody complexes and resultant disorders such as erythema nodosum. A "clear" zone between infiltrate and overlying epidermis is characteristic of lepromatous leprosy, unlike the encroachment on basal epidermis of the tuberculoid infiltrate.

44. The answer is D. *(Anderson, 9/e. pp 2–3.)* The cytoplasmic matrix contains numerous organelles with highly specialized functions. Whereas mitochondria are the "power" units of the cell involved with the Krebs cycle and anaerobic metabolism, the endoplasmic reticulum is a complex network of rodlike tubules containing ribosomes and is involved in protein synthesis (rough endoplasmic reticulum). Lysosomes are round bodies containing enzymes involved in inflammation. These include the sulfatases, desoxyribonucleases, hydrolases, and acid phosphatases. The Golgi apparatus (complex) is made up of tiny vesicles, membranes, and vacuoles and is also involved in protein synthesis, as it receives the synthesized proteins from the endoplasmic reticulum. The Golgi complex appears to collect, segregate, and export protein. Microbodies are membrane-bound spheres that contain catalase and oxidases. Epithelial cells, especially surface-lining cells, are held together by connections referred to as intercellular junctions. Desmosomes (squamous cells), tight junctions (zonula occludens), and gap junctions (nexuses) are examples of such membrane connectors.

45. The answer is E. *(Robbins, 4/e. pp 365–366, 372.)* Lymphogranuloma venereum, usually transmitted by sexual contact, is caused by obligate intracellular parasites that contain both RNA and DNA and belong to the genus *Chlamydia (C. trachomatis)*. Chlamydial agents, originally thought to be viruses because they form inclusion bodies in infected cells, also cause trachoma, inclusion conjunctivitis, and psittacosis-ornithosis. The other infections listed are caused by spirochetes and are nonvenereal.

46. The answer is E. *(Henry, 18/e. pp 452–454.)* Elevations in cerebrospinal fluid globulins often occur in multiple sclerosis and other demyelinating diseases. An abnormal band on electrophoresis may occur even in the absence of elevated globulins. Late tertiary syphilis may cause these findings, but they would not occur in the secondary stage. Tumor or meningeal leukemia can also produce elevated levels of globulin in cerebrospinal fluid, but the presence of tumor cells and absence of an electrophoretic band would lead to the proper diagnosis.

47. The answer is C. *(Robbins, 4/e. pp 527–530.)* Hemolytic disease of the newborn is characterized by anemia, jaundice, tissue edema, and hepatosplenomegaly. The transmission of maternal antibody (transplacental transmission) causes the disease because of incompatibility between maternal and fetal blood types. ABO incompatibilities occur often but are not severe; however, both ABO and Rh antigens may cause the disease. There are many Rh antigens that do not cause disease, but RhD is the usual antigen causing mild to very severe disease, except in the first pregnancy. The frequency increases with repeat pregnancies as antibody level rises, and anti-RhD IgG must be given to a nonsensitized Rh-negative mother within 72 h of delivery or termination (abortion) of the first and of all subsequent pregnancies.

48. The answer is A. *(Robbins, 4/e. p 240.)* All tumors whether benign or malignant have a supporting stroma composed of varying amounts of connective tissue and blood supply. The cellularity can range from that of a highly cellular lesion, such as oat cell carcinoma of the lung or Burkitt's lymphoma, to that of a relatively hypocellular lesion, such as a hyalinized neurilemmoma, but the cellularity of the tumor per se does not usually influence the texture. Firmness and even hardness of tumors are a function of the amount of collagenous stroma present. The term *desmoplasia* refers to a collagenized and fibroblastic stroma; an example is carcinoma of the breast, which has the texture of a water chestnut because of the concurrent proliferation of the fibrous stroma with the carcinoma. Tumors that lack a collagenized fibrous stroma tend to be softer regardless of the tumor cellularity per se. Malignant tumors of mesenchyme have a fleshy character because of very little connective tissue stroma; examples include fibrosarcoma, liposarcoma, and leiomyosarcoma. There are a few exceptions to the desmoplastic rule, and an obvious example is a tumor of cartilage in which the hyaline cartilage matrix accounts for the firmness; some chondrosarcomas, however, may be soft and friable.

49. The answer is B. *(Robbins, 4/e. pp 695, 1070.)* A fulminating septic state should always be considered and excluded whenever the constellation of fever, deteriorating mental status, skin hemorrhages, and shock develops. Such conditions can be seen in gram-negative rod septicemia caused by any of the coliforms (gram-negative endotoxic shock) or fulminant meningococcemia (Waterhouse-Friderichsen syndrome). However, a form of nonbacterial vasculitis termed *thrombotic thrombocytopenic purpura (TTP)* is notorious for producing a clinical syndrome very similar to fulminating infective states. It is characterized by arteriole and capillary occlusions by fibrin and platelet microthrombi and is usually unassociated with any of the predisposing states seen in disseminated intravascular coagulopathy (DIC), such as malignancy, infection, retained fetus, and amniotic fluid embolism. Macrocytic hemolytic anemia, variable jaundice, renal failure, skin hemorrhages, and central nervous system dysfunction are all seen in TTP and are related to the fibrin thrombi, which can be demonstrated with skin, bone marrow, and lymph node biopsies. The vasculitis usually shows no inflammatory cells, which distinguishes TTP from other forms of vasculitis. There is less coagulopathy in TTP than is found in DIC, and hemolytic anemia is generally not found in idiopathic or autoimmune thrombocytopenic purpura. The condition of patients with TTP may be temporarily improved by plasmapheresis, but the outcome is usually grim.

50. The answer is C. *(Henry, 18/e. pp 76–77.)* The type of blood sample sent to the laboratory, the type of container used to collect blood, the manner in which the blood specimen was collected, and the preparation of the patient (appropriate fasting, drug history, exercise) prior to venipuncture are just as important to the final laboratory result as the analytic method used by the laboratory to arrive at the result. All these factors can cause deviations in laboratory results, and they should be considered before accepting abnormal laboratory results. Red blood cells can readily lyse because of alcohol left on the arm while swabbing the skin, use of unclean or poorly dried syringes or too large a needle bore (17 gauge, for example), or a traumatic venipuncture. Since red blood cells contain a higher concentration of K^+ than does serum or plasma, even moderate hemolysis of red cells can cause spurious elevation of serum K^+. If the serum clot tube is seen to be slightly pink, most laboratories will notify the ward that an improper sample has been obtained. Once the laboratory result is confirmed as being valid, the next step is to exclude intravascular hemolysis within the patient before making a diagnosis of hyperkalemia.

51. The answer is C. *(Henry, 18/e. pp 154–155. Robbins, 4/e. pp 1242–1243.)* Parathyroid hormone (PTH), by affecting the kidneys, bones, and intestinal mucosa, is the principal regulator of plasma levels of phosphate and calcium. PTH, by its action on renal tubular cells, not only causes decreased phosphate reabsorption, it causes increased calcium reabsorption; these reciprocal processes result in a decrease in serum phosphate and a corresponding increase in extracellular calcium levels. Extracellular levels of calcium are also maintained by the release of calcium during PTH-induced osteocytic and osteoclastic osteolysis, a process that is regarded as the mobilization of calcium from bone. PTH also may induce the intestinal mucosa to absorb calcium derived from dietary sources.

52. The answer is A. *(Henry, 18/e. pp 264–265, 276–278.)* Serum glutamic-oxaloacetic transaminase (SGOT) levels (curve II) become elevated within 12 h after nearly all acute myocardial infarctions; they generally reach a peak level within 48 h and return to normal within 4 to 5 days. After myocardial infarctions, creatine phosphokinase levels (curve I) rise and fall more rapidly than do SGOT levels. Lactic dehydrogenase levels (curve III) also become elevated within 1 day after infarctions, but they remain elevated for about 10 days. Alkaline phosphatase and 5'-nucleotidase levels, normal during infarctions, usually show marked increases in patients who have obstructive jaundice.

53. The answer is D. *(Henry, 18/e. pp 42–43, 125.)* Although most laboratories are capable of directly measuring the serum or urine osmolality with accurate osmometers, it is useful to remember the following formula:

$$\text{Osmolality (mosmol/kg) } H_2O = 2 \times [Na^+] + \frac{[\text{glucose}]}{20} + \frac{[\text{BUN}]}{3}$$

This formula gives an approximation of the serum osmolality in a given patient, since Na^+, glucose, and BUN account for at least 95 percent of the dissolved solutes composing the osmolality. The normal serum osmolality falls within the range of 285 to 310 mosmol/kg H_2O. An often overlooked cause of profound water loss with dehydration (in osmotic diseases) in elderly diabetic patients is nonketotic, hypersomolar coma. These patients enter a phase of coma and dehydration with vascular collapse owing to hypovolemia caused by profound osmotic diuresis that is in turn due to the striking hyperglycemia. The serum acetoacetic acid and ketone levels may be normal or mildly elevated in contrast to the ketoacidosis of diabetic coma in younger patients.

54. The answer is E. *(Wilson, 12/e. pp 1369–1371, 1374–1375.)* An elevated serum amylase level is usually associated with acute pancreatitis; it is practically diagnostic if it is more than three times normal, and if salivary gland disease and intestinal perforation or infarction are excluded. There may be increased amylase with parotitis alone, but increased lipase (more sensitive and much more specific) only with pancreatitis. Elevated amylase may be associated with renal disease because of decreased clearance and with morphine administration because of decreased excretion. Low serum amylase has been noted with serum protein loss in congestive heart failure. Amylase can be produced by certain tumors (lung, breast, ovarian cancer). In these and in acidotic states, the amylase must be distinguished from that of pancreatitis by isoenzyme analysis. P isoamylases arise from the pancreas; S isoamylases arise from nonpancreatic sources, as in diabetic ketoacidosis.

55. The answer is D. *(Grizzle, Arch Pathol Lab Med 113:727–728, 1989.)* In Cushing's syndrome diagnostic laboratory tests have improved from relatively nonspecific urinary assays of 17-ketogenic steroids and 17-hydroxycorticosteroids to more specific radioimmunoassays measuring ACTH, corticotropin releasing factor (CRF), cortisol, and other plasma steroids as well as urinary free cortisol—a reliable, cost-effective screening method. After diagnosis of Cushing's syndrome, its cause must be identified by the dexamethasone (synthetic analogue of cortisol) high-dose suppression test, reliable ACTH radioimmunoassays, and imaging techniques of computed tomography (sella turcica) and nuclear magnetic resonance. Small pituitary microadenomas may be identified now by selective venous sampling for ACTH and other peptides from the inferior petrosal sinuses draining the pituitary. Plasma cortisol levels fluctuate rather widely and the urinary 17-ketosteroids give information about androgen metabolites, not about glucocorticoid activity.

56. The answer is D. *(Henry, 18/e. pp 241–243, 260–262, 697.)* In polycythemia vera the serum alkaline phosphatase level is not increased. However, the neutrophil alkaline phosphatase is markedly elevated in 80 percent of patients with polycythemia vera, while this leukocyte alkaline phosphatase level is depressed in chronic myelogenous leukemia. Serum alkaline phosphatase is usually quite markedly elevated in such hepatobiliary diseases as obstructive jaundice, intrahepatic cholestasis, biliary cirrhosis, and infectious mononucleosis. Milder elevations occur in alcoholic cirrhosis and viral hepatitis. The placental alkaline phosphatase isoenzyme peaks during the third trimester and returns to normal post partum.

57. The answer is A. *(Henry, 18/e. pp 120–121.)* The renal plasma clearance of any substance *(X)* is expressed as the volume of plasma from which X is removed by renal activity per unit of time, usually 1 min. In the clearance formula shown below, U_x represents the concentration of X in milligrams per milliliter of urine; V represents urine volume per minute and usually is derived from a 24-h urine volume; P_x represents the plasma concentration of X in milligrams per milliliter; and C_x represents the volume of plasma cleared of substance X per minute.

$$C_x = \frac{(U_x)(V)}{P_x}$$

By interpolation of the given data into appropriate units and by substitution, the equation becomes

$$C_x = \frac{(0.469 \text{ mg/mL})(0.535 \text{ mL/min})}{0.02 \text{ mg/mL}}$$

The answer is 12.5 mL/min. For males, normal creatinine clearance values range from 107 to 139 mL/min; for females, the range is 87 to 107 mL/min.

58. The answer is C. *(Bullough, pp 5.4–5.8.)* Hyperuricemia, prominent in gout, occurs most often secondary to disorders that increase production or reduce excretion of uric acid. These include myeloproliferative disorders and some cancers in which there is increased turnover of nucleic acid, with resultant hyperuricemia. Reduced excretion of uric acid may arise from renal causes, or from competition by certain organic acids, as in starvation ketosis. Chondrocalcinosis, or calcium pyrophosphate dihydrate (CPPD) deposition disease, is not associated with hyperuricemia.

59. The answer is A. *(Robbins, 4/e. pp 323–325.)* If bilirubinuria and pyridium therapy are excluded, the presence of pink-orange-brown casts with contained granular debris or intact red cells within the casts always implies the presence of significant glomerular damage, usually in the form of immune complex glomerulonephritis (poststreptococcal, lupus, Goodpasture's) or owing to renal infarction. Damage to the glomerular capillary loops or the basement membrane allows the leakage of red cells and protein, which condense into casts in the distal tubules, are subsequently passed into the urine, and become directly visible under the microscope in urinalysis. Whereas renal biopsies are usually necessary to categorize the nature of the glomerulonephritis completely, poststreptococcal glomerulonephritis may be implicated if the antistreptolysin O (ASO) titer or anti-DNAase-B titers are elevated.

60. The answer is B. *(Robbins, 4/e. pp 243–250.)* As all medical oncologists and students of oncology are painfully aware, tumors do not read textbooks and cannot be expected to follow predicted courses in every clinical circumstance. Thus, many exceptions and deviations from the expected occur. An important predictor of a given tumor's behavior, however, is the differentiation, which is a histologic parameter that gives some index as to the degree of resemblance of the tumor to the cell of origin; that is, differentiation states to what degree the tumor resembles its parent cell or tissues. Well-differentiated tumors resemble their cells of origin to a great extent, while poorly differentiated tumors do not resemble their origins to an appreciable extent. With some exceptions tumors may be expected to behave according to their differentiation. Furthermore, the growth rate of tumors appears to correlate with their level of differentiation, with the less-differentiated tumors growing faster than well-differentiated ones. The term *grade* implies differentiation and in some cases may be synonymous; for example, grade I tumors are well differentiated, while grade III tumors are poorly differentiated. Higher grade tumors tend to have more mitoses, which generally correlate with aggressiveness and poorer outcome.

61. The answer is B. *(Wilson, 12/e. pp 553–555, 563.)* The pneumococcus *(Streptococcus pneumoniae)* is a gram-positive, encapsulated coccus, differentiated from other alpha-hemolytic streptococci by bile solubility or serologic typing. But inhibition of pneumococci by Optochin is easier and has about 90 percent specificity. Capsular polysaccharides form the basis for division into serotypes; when exposed to type-specific antisera they show a positive precipitin reaction or capsular swelling, the quellung reaction. Detection of pneumococcal capsular polysaccharides in sputum or body fluids by immunologic methods (CIE or latex agglutination) are other methods for presumptive diagnosis of infection, but cross reactions between pneumococci and other bacteria occur. So, immunologic diagnosis is less specific than bacteriologic diagnosis by capsular typing by the quellung reaction. Capsular polysaccharides protect pneumococci from phagocytosis and are virulence factors. M protein occurs in the cell walls of pathogenic group A beta-hemolytic streptococci *(S. pyogenes)* and functions as the principal virulence factor by inhibiting phagocytosis.

62. The answer is C. *(Henry, 18/e. pp 745–747.)* Von Willebrand's disease is not as rare as once thought, and numerous subtypes, which are delineated by two-dimensional electrophoresis, have been described. The disease is characterized clinically by mucocutaneous bleeding, menorrhagia, and epistaxis. Milder forms of the disease may not be diagnosed until the patient is older. Factor VIII is a complex of several components that can be discerned electrophoretically. Of all the factor VIII components, factor VIII:R, or ristocetin cofactor, is most apt to be abnormal in von Willebrand's disease. The coagulant (C) and the related antigen (Ag) forms of factor VIII may sometimes be normal in various autosomal dominant types. Most patients even with the milder forms will have decreased factor VIII:R. Prothrombin time and fibrinogen levels are not affected in this disorder.

63. The answer is A. *(Henry, 18/e. pp 266–270.)* The patient described probably has hepatitis, according to the values given for the five isoenzymes of lactic dehydrogenase (LDH). Liver cells contain higher proportions of LDH_4 and LDH_5 than do myocardium or red blood cells, both of which contain greater relative amounts of LDH_1 and LDH_2. Lung tissue is high in LDH_3, and brain tissue contains only small amounts of LDH_5.

64. The answer is B. *(Robbins, 4/e. pp 253, 261, 288, 715–716, 718.)* Burkitt's lymphoma is one of the most rapidly growing tumors known to oncologists. Most tumors grow without inhibition by means of a decrease in the time spent within the cell growth cycle itself, a reduction in the total numbers of cells dying, or many more stable cells leaving G_0 to enter the cycle at G_1. One or all of these mechanisms may be in effect, along with a lack of inhibition of cell growth. Such inhibition is not completely understood, but cells are known to be delayed in progressing to mitosis from G_2. Permanent cells are essentially nondividing and usually die. In African Burkitt's lymphoma, but not necessarily in American Burkitt's lymphoma, high titers of serum antibody to Epstein-Barr viral capsid antigen have been described, along with incorporation of the viral genome. A translocation occurs between chromosome 8 (site of proto-oncogene c-*myc*) and chromosome 14, which carries the heavy-chain Ig gene, t (8;14).

65. The answer is D. *(Robbins, 4/e. pp 269, 272.)* The association of the chemical and physical environment (with its implied hazards of toxic wastes, mainly from industrial pollution) with the development of tumors in humans is becoming a specialized field in itself. Major legislation and public health efforts are just beginning to place emphasis on these hazards. A major clue to the implication of environmental factors lies in the clustering of rare tumor types in populations in which such an incidence is unexpected. For example, cases of angiosarcoma of the liver (a relatively rare tumor) were identified in employees of a rubber company and in a few residents living near the plant where the monomer vinyl chloride was present in the atmosphere. Exposure to asbestos in shipyard, roofing, and insulation workers has led to the development of not only pleural and peritoneal malignant mesotheliomas, but solid malignant tumors of the lung and viscera as well. Although it increases the risk of tuberculosis, silicosis has not, by itself, increased the risk of developing cancer. Similarly, beryllium vapor (from the manufacture of alloys, ceramics, high-technology electronics, and fluorescent light bulbs) causes marked granulomatous disease but has not been identified as a carcinogen. Cyanide is lethal if ingested. Carbon tetrachloride and chloroform may cause hepatic necrosis and are potentially lethal, but neither is implicated in tumorigenesis. Foundry workers are at risk of developing pulmonary and nasal sinus cancers when they are regularly exposed to nickel or chromium compounds.

66. The answer is D. *(Henry, 18/e. pp 314–317.)* Triiodothyronine (T_3) is the thyroid hormone with the greatest physiologic activity, although thyroxine (T_4) is present in greater quantities and thus is usually the best measure of thyroid activity. Monoiodotyrosine (MIT) and diiodotyrosine (DIT) are not released from the gland and have little activity. Thyroglobulin is the carrier protein for binding stored thyroid hormones.

67. The answer is C. *(Robbins, 4/e. pp 1260–1261.)* A tendency to lose salt and water often appears in adrenogenital syndrome with adrenocortical hyperplasia. There is general agreement that in the salt-losing form of this syndrome, aldosterol and cortisol production is deficient, a consequence of genetically impaired biosynthesis of adrenal corticoids. Adrenogenital syndrome also may be known as "congenital virilizing adrenocortical hyperplasia," a generic term that probably should be discarded because it paradoxically includes forms not associated with virilization.

68. The answer is A. *(Robbins, 4/e. pp 876–878.)* Celiac disease (gluten-sensitive enteropathy) is a disorder characterized by malabsorption induced by sensitivity to the gluten and gliadin in certain cereals, especially wheat, rye, and barley. Exposure to gluten results in a typical malabsorption syndrome of varying severity. There is a high incidence of HLA-B8 (over 85 percent of cases) and HLA-Dw3 (over 90 percent) antigens. Characteristic morphological changes include villous atrophy, crypt hypertrophy with increased mitotic activity in crypts, and chronic inflammatory infiltrate in the lamina propria of the duodenum and jejunum. The *proximal* small intestine shows the most severe and extensive involvement. Immunocytes express surface IgA antigliadin antibodies. Antigliadin antibodies are also present in the serum but the level correlates poorly with clinical status. Complications are numerous and, with disease lasting 10 years or more, include a 10 to 15 percent risk of malignancy. Half of these cancers are B-cell lymphomas; the remainder are carcinomas that may arise anywhere in the gastrointestinal tract, but occur frequently in the small bowel.

69. The answer is B. *(Robbins, 4/e. pp 52, 140–144, 530–536.)* Familial hypercholesterolemia (FH) is a common autosomal dominant (AD) disorder caused by mutation in the low-density lipoprotein (LDL) receptor gene located on chromosome 19. These gene mutations impair LDL transport and catabolism, with accumulation of LDL cholesterol in plasma. Elevated cholesterol levels result in skin xanthomas, early atherosclerosis, and increased risk of myocardial infarction. There is absent or deficient LDL receptor activity in homozygotes and one-half normal receptor activity in heterozygotes. CF is a fairly common AR disorder in whites (1:2500). Exocrine glands produce viscous mucus and sweat with high sodium and chloride concentration. The mutant gene product is unknown but the CF gene is localized on the long arm of chromosome 7. CF is manifest clinically only in homozygotes; parents are asymptomatic heterozygous carriers of the trait. PKU is an AR disorder of amino acid metabolism due to mutation in the gene coding for phenylalanine hydroxylase. Chromosome location is 12 and six different mutations are known. Myeloperoxidase deficiency has a frequency of 1:2000; slow bacterial killing is the major problem. Alkaptonuria is rare, the mutant gene product is homogentisic acid oxidase, and abnormal pigmentation of connective tissue (ochronosis) will result. *brown or grey discoloration*

70. The answer is C. *(Robbins, 4/e. p 127.)* Any deviation from the normal number of chromosomes, from their normal structure, or any combination of the two is an aberration that, if unbalanced, is termed *aneuploidy*. If the alterations remain balanced (balanced translocations), the condition is termed *euploidy*. Aneuploidy can result from the addition of a single chromosome to a pair (trisomy) or from translocations, inversions, duplications, and deletions.

71. The answer is A. *(Wilson, 12/e. pp 1199–1200.)* Renal tubular acidosis (RTA) can be either due to a gradient defect (the classic form) or due to bicarbonate wastage. In the classic form of this syndrome, too many hydrogen ions diffuse back from tubular urine to blood. This "back-diffusion" occurs in the distal tubules and prevents the formation of a steep pH gradient between blood and tubular urine. Ammonia excretion is normal in both forms of RTA. In RTA caused by bicarbonate wastage, the depressed reabsorption of bicarbonate ions in the proximal tubules leads to the spillage of these ions into urine.

72. The answer is D. *(Robbins, 4/e. pp 342, 782.)* Most cases of lobar pneumonia are caused by *Streptococcus pneumoniae* (reclassification of the pneumococcus). Streptococcal or pneumococcal pneumonia involves one or more lobes and is often seen in alcoholics or debilitated persons. Type 3 pneumococcus *(S. pneumoniae)* causes a virulent lobar pneumonia characterized by mucoid sputum, which is also seen in *Klebsiella* pneumonia. *K. pneumoniae* (Friedländer's bacillus) usually produces a bronchopneumonia, rather than lobar pneumonia, but is clinically indistinguishable from pneumococcal lobar pneumonia. *Legionella* species cause a fibrinopurulent lobular pneumonia that tends to be confluent, almost appearing lobar.

73. The answer is E. *(Wilson, 12/e. p 1829.)* The porphyrias are inherited or acquired disorders of heme biosynthesis with varied patterns of overproduction, accumulation, and excretion of heme synthesis intermediates. Major characteristics include intermittent neurologic dysfunction and skin sensitivity to sunlight, but intermittent acute porphyria shows no skin photosensitivity, unlike the other types. Porphyria cutanea tarda is the most common type and has chronic skin lesions (face, forehead, forearms) and frequent hepatic disease. Excess urinary porphobilinogen excretion occurs in variegate porphyria and intermittent acute porphyria. Detection of porphobilinogen in the urine forms the basis for a positive Watson-Schwartz reaction in the diagnosis of variegate and intermittent acute porphyria.

74. The answer is D. *(Robbins, 4/e. pp 165–167.)* B cells possess surface membrane IgM and IgD, with monomeric IgM the antigen receptor of all B cells. B cells also express the pan–B-cell antigens CD19 and CD20, which is obviously of practical value in differentiating a chronic leukemia such as chronic lymphocytic leukemia (CLL) in which transformed B cells possess surface IgM and IgD and express CD19 and CD20 antigens, but not the early B cell antigen CD10. In contrast, CD8 and CD4 are on 30 percent and 60 percent of peripheral T cells, respectively. CD4 is a marker for T helper cells, and CD8 a marker for cytotoxic/suppressor T cells. B lymphocytes have receptors for fixed complement components C3b and C3d and for the Fc portion of IgG. Immunologic diagnosis of B-cell lymphoid tumors by immunofluorescence or flow cytometry shows the cell surface immunoglobulins and cluster differentiation antigens through detection by monoclonal antibodies; molecular biology techniques reveal Ig gene rearrangements on the altered B cells.

75. The answer is D. *(Robbins, 4/e. pp 357–358.)* *Yersinia* (formerly called *Pasteurella*) is an important genus of gram-negative bacilli that causes a wide variety of human and animal disease, ranging from plague *(Y. pestis)* to acute mesenteric lymphadenitis *(Y. enterocolitica)* in older children and young adults. *Y. enterocolitica* infections also occur in the terminal ileum in young adults, causing an ileitis that produces inflammation not unlike that seen in some stages of Crohn's disease (regional enteritis). Since the organisms grow slowly on enrichment media, they may be overgrown by other coliforms at 37°C. The organisms may be isolated by means of cold enhancement at 4°C.

76. The answer is B. *(Robbins, 4/e. pp 182–183.)* Delayed-hypersensitivity reactions are mediated by T lymphocytes and other mononuclear cells. The reaction requires previous exposure to antigen, frequently a large protein, and takes from 1 to 3 days to develop fully. Only true palpable induration is considered a positive reaction.

77. The answer is C. *(Robbins, 4/e. pp 386–387, 393–394.)* In the approximate center of the photomicrograph is the classic, refractile, double-walled spherule of the deep fungus *Coccidioides immitis,* which is several times the diameter of the largest inflammatory cell nearby. Coccidioidomycosis is endemic in California, Arizona, New Mexico, and parts of Nevada, Utah, and Texas, where it resides in the arid soils and is contracted by direct inhalation of airborne dust. If inhaled, it produces a primary pulmonary infection that is usually benign and self-limiting in immunologically competent persons, often with several days of fever and upper respiratory flulike symptoms. However, certain ethnic groups, such as some blacks, Asians, and Filipinos, are at risk of developing a potentially lethal disseminated form of the disease that can involve the central nervous system. If the large, double-walled spherule containing numerous endospores can be demonstrated outside the lungs (e.g., in a skin biopsy), this is evidence of dissemination. Antibodies of high titers are detectable by means of complement fixation studies in patients undergoing spontaneous recovery. Amphotericin B is usually reserved for treating high-risk and disseminated infection. The cultured mycelia of the organism on Sabouraud's agar present a hazard for laboratory workers.

78. The answer is A. *(Robbins, 4/e. pp 151–153, 665.)* The glycogen storage diseases are due to defective metabolism of glycogen, and at least eleven syndromes from genetic defects in the responsible enzymes have been described. Most of these glycogenoses are inherited as autosomal recessive disorders. Von Gierke's disease (type I) results from deficiency of glucose-6-phospha-tase, the hepatic enzyme needed for conversion of G6P to glucose, with glycogen accumulation particularly in the enlarged liver and kidney and hypoglycemia. Diagnosis requires biopsy demonstration of excess liver glycogen plus either absent or low liver G6P activity, or a diabetic glucose tolerance curve, or hyperuricemia. Von Gierke's disease is the major hepatic or hepatorenal type of glycogenosis. Lysosomal glucosidase deficiency causes Pompe's disease (type II). Glycogen storage is widespread but most prominent in the heart (cardiomegaly). In brancher glycogenosis (type IV) there is accumulation of amylopectin or abnormal glycogen in liver, heart, skeletal muscle, and brain. The major myopathic form, McArdle's disease (type V), is due to lack of muscle phosphorylase. Glucose-6-phosphate dehydrogenase (G6PD) deficiency may cause oxidant-induced hemolytic anemia. The gene is X-linked recessive. One variant is present in about 10 percent of American blacks.

79. The answer is C. *(Robbins, 4/e. pp 373–375.)* Pathogenic mycobacteria, including *M. tuberculosis,* have a known propensity for resistance to drying in the environment, survival for extended periods of time on inanimate surfaces, resistance to alkali and acids, and impermeability to routine tissue and Gram stains. Many of these features are thought to be related to the very high lipid and wax content of the bacilli, which makes up some 60 percent of the total dry weight. Mycolic acid is only one of many fatty acids present. Virulence is thought to be related to the presence of the mycoside trehalose 6-6 dimycolate (cord factor).

80. The answer is A. *(Robbins, 4/e. pp 312–315, 320, 325.)* Togaviruses, a family of helical, predominantly single-stranded RNA viruses, include dengue and yellow fever viruses (both associated with hemorrhagic fever) and eastern, western, and St. Louis encephalitis viruses. These are all arthropod-borne. The causative agent of epidemic hemorrhagic keratoconjunctivitis is usually the type B adenovirus, an icosahedral double-stranded DNA virus. Herpes simplex keratoconjunctivitis, although frequently recurrent, is not epidemic.

81. The answer is E. *(Robbins, 4/e. pp 374–375.)* *Mycobacterium tuberculosis* is an obligate aerobe—thus its predilection for pulmonary infection. The high content of lipids in its cell wall is in part responsible for its acid-fast response to Ziehl-Neelsen staining. The frequency of occurrence of drug-resistant mutants in this organism has necessitated simultaneous use of multiple chemotherapeutic agents against it. Persons with silicosis have a high incidence of infection with *M. tuberculosis,* which on culture requires several weeks to grow.

82. The answer is D. *(Robbins, 4/e. pp 774, 796–797.)* Drug-induced respiratory changes include bronchospasm, pulmonary edema, hypersensitivity pneumonitis, and chronic pneumonitis with fibrosis. Amiodarone, given for ventricular tachycardia, is concentrated in the lung and causes pneumonitis, with resultant fibrosis in 5 to 15 percent of patients. The cytotoxic drug bleomycin, used in cancer chemotherapy, also causes pneumonitis and fibrosis because of direct drug toxicity and stimulation of inflammatory cells to infiltrate alveoli. Methotrexate, another cytotoxic anticancer agent that inhibits synthesis of DNA, and nitrofurantoin both may cause hypersensitivity pneumonitis. Very small doses of aspirin may cause asthmatic attacks and urticaria in patients with rhinitis and nasal polyps. In these patients, aspirin probably inhibits the cyclooxygenase path of arachidonic acid metabolism with no effect on the lipoxygenase path, so that decreased prostaglandins, increased bronchoconstrictor leukotrienes, and asthma result. In acute salicylate poisoning, the initial event is respiratory stimulation with loss of carbon dioxide.

83. The answer is C. *(Robbins, 4/e. pp 318–324.)* Influenza is caused by small RNA viruses, classified as myxoviruses. All the other viral illnesses listed in the question are caused by herpesviruses, which are relatively large, double-stranded DNA viruses. Shingles and chickenpox are caused by herpes zoster, which is identical to varicella. Cytomegalovirus causes cytomegalic inclusion disease, and Epstein-Barr (EB) virus causes mononucleosis.

84. The answer is E. *(Robbins, 4/e. pp 333–334, 784–785.)* *Mycoplasma pneumoniae,* the causative agent of primary atypical interstitial pneumonia, belongs to the mycoplasma group of tiny pleuropneumonia-like organisms (PPLOs, or Eaton agents), which lack cell walls and are beyond the resolution of light microscopy. *M. pneumoniae* can cause up to 50 percent of pneumonias in college students and mainly affects adolescents and young adults. The interstitial pneumonia with mononuclear response is similar to viral pneumonia; pharyngitis and tracheobronchitis with persistent cough are common. Serum immunoglobulins that agglutinate human type O red cells at 4°C (cold agglutinins) are often present; this test is nonspecific but suggestive of *M. pneumoniae.*

85. The answer is C. *(Robbins, 4/e. pp 488–489.)* Despite current controversy, most researchers agree that women taking oral contraceptives are at risk, however small, of developing myocardial infarction, especially if the woman is a cigarette smoker, and vascular thrombi that may lead to strokes and pulmonary embolism and infarction. Also very minimal in terms of numbers of cases are hepatic adenomas, which have been recorded in patients taking oral estrogens over a protracted period of time. Conflicting evidence is found concerning the risk of developing endometrial carcinoma. Some researchers have shown a definite risk of developing uterine cancer, but not all series have demonstrated a positive correlation. The same problem exists in estimation of the risk of developing breast cancer. Vaginal adenosis develops not in the women taking estrogens themselves, but rather in the female offspring of mothers who received diethylstilbestrol (DES) while pregnant. Some of these daughters have also developed clear cell carcinoma of the cervix, an adenocarcinoma that carries a rather poor prognosis. DES binds to cell nuclear DNA and hence may act as a cocarcinogen rather than as a mere promoter.

86. The answer is D. (*Robbins, 4/e. pp 490–492.*) The seemingly innumerable deleterious effects of alcohol abuse are recognized as constituting a major public health problem even in non-Western locations, such as Africa and Asia. The effects may be socioeconomic (divorce, absenteeism, and high insurance rates due to automobile accidents), political, moral, or organic. Indeed, it is difficult to think of an organ or organ system that does not develop a physical dysfunction, either reversible or irreversible, in response to excessive intake of ethanol. Subdural hematomas are commonly seen in alcoholics. Portal vein thrombosis is rarely seen in the absence of nutritional or Laënnec's cirrhosis. Levels of the muscle and cardiac enzyme creatine phosphokinase may be elevated in states of alcoholic myocardiosis, cardiomyopathy, alcoholic rhabdomyolysis, or trauma to skeletal muscles while the patient is in an alcoholic toxic state. Primary biliary cirrhosis occurs predominantly in middle-aged women and its etiology is unknown, although marked immunologic factors have been described, as well as marked copper deposition in the liver, with normal serum ceruloplasmin.

87. The answer is C. (*Robbins, 4/e. p 362.*) Listeriosis is a food-borne illness (e.g., via milk products, coleslaw) usually occurring in the immunocompromised, in pregnant women and their fetuses, and in the debilitated elderly. *Listeria monocytogenes* is a gram-positive, motile bacillus, often found within circulating lymphocytes (similar to *Legionella*). Maternal infection is mild; fetal infection is severe. Meningitis is predominant in neonatal infections and in opportunistic adult disease, and *Listeria monocytogenes* is responsible for about 2 percent of bacterial meningitis cases in this country. True epithelioid granulomas are rare, although macrophages may appear late, following neutrophil infiltration or abscesses in organs or lymph nodes.

88. The answer is D. *(Wilson, 12/e. pp 1402–1409.)* AIDS is caused by infection with the retrovirus human immunodeficiency virus (HIV) (formerly called HTLV III/LAV). The virus infects T helper cells, preventing function, destroying cells, and increasing susceptibility to and incidence of infection. Cytotoxic/suppressor T cells may be normal, slightly increased, or decreased in number, although they show a proportional increase in comparison to helper T cells, which are markedly decreased. In AIDS, the ratio of helper to suppressor cells is inverted, being approximately 1:2, instead of the normal 2:1. Wide defects of immune function in AIDS include defects in natural killer cells, in monocytes, and in virus-specific cytotoxic T cells and B cells. B cells are polyclonally activated, resulting in hypergammaglobulinemia. Histologic diagnosis of chronic lymphoid interstitial pneumonitis in a child under 13 years of age is indicative of AIDS unless tests for HIV are negative.

89. The answer is B. *(Robbins, 4/e. pp 294–296, 798–801.)* Small cell lung cancer (SCLC) is usually a central or hilar tumor, although the rare combined (small cell plus squamous or adenocarcinoma) type often occurs in the lung periphery. The abnormal cells shown are usually in tight clusters with nuclear molding in both sputum specimens and tissue sections, whereas leukemic cells are smaller, more rounded, and not in clusters but scattered singly throughout the specimen. Ultrastructurally, some SCLC cells show neurosecretory granules, and immunohistochemical stains are usually positive for neuroendocrine markers (neuron-specific enolase, chromogranin A). Both SCLC and bronchial carcinoids are considered to be neuroendocrine lung tumors, although other non-SCLC tumors of the lung can also express neuroendocrine markers. Paraneoplastic syndromes produced by these cells include inappropriate ADH/AVP release, which causes hyponatremia owing to excess water reabsorption; ACTH release resulting in Cushing's syndrome; or serotonin release with the carcinoid syndrome—episodic facial flushing, vasomotor responses, and bronchoconstriction. It should be noted that no specimen, whether cytologic or histologic, should *ever* be submitted without relevant history.

90. The answer is B. *(Robbins, 4/e. pp 441–447.)* Vitamin D is essential for maintenance of normal bone remodeling in the adult; therefore, a significant deficiency in adults leads to poorly mineralized bone, or osteomalacia. Deficiency also results in decreased intestinal absorption of calcium, inadequate serum calcium and phosphorus, and, therefore, impaired mineralization of osteoid. Defective mineralization of osteoid causes formation of soft, easily deformed bones. Since there is no decreased production of osteoid matrix, a relative excess of woven bone or osteoid with wide osteoid seams results.

91. The answer is D. *(Robbins, 4/e. pp 65–68.)* Granulomatous inflammation is characterized by the presence of granulomas, consisting of 1- to 2-mm foci of modified macrophages (epithelioid cells) surrounded by mononuclear cells, mainly lymphocytes. It is a chronic inflammation initiated by a variety of infectious and noninfectious agents. Indigestible organisms or particles, or T cell–mediated immunity to the inciting agent, or both, appear essential for formation of granulomas. Although tuberculosis is the classic infectious granulomatous disease, several other infectious disorders are characterized by formation of granulomas, including deep fungal infections (coccidioidomycosis and histoplasmosis), schistosomiasis, syphilis, brucellosis, lymphogranuloma venereum, and cat-scratch disease. In sarcoidosis, a disease of unknown cause, the granulomas are noncaseating, which may assist in histologic differentiation from tuberculosis.

92. The answer is A. *(Robbins, 4/e. pp 301–302.)* The photomicrograph in the question shows an immunoperoxidase reaction, a technique fostered by Sternberger in the early 1970s to identify antigens within cells by the use of an antibody specific for the antigen sought. Following incubation with a specific antibody directed against the target antigen (primary antibody incubation), a secondary antibody incubation is conducted using heterologous immune sera directed against the first antibody. For example, the primary antibody may be rabbit antihuman IgG. If human IgG is present on or within a given cell, binding occurs. Secondary antibody could then be goat antirabbit, which now binds to the rabbit IgG. Then horseradish peroxidase-antiperoxidase conjugate is applied, which links to the antibody complexes. The last step is a chromogen substrate, in this case rust-brown diaminobenzidine. Rust-brown granules indicate a positive reaction. This useful technique (or a modification of it, such as the use of highly specific and sensitive monoclonal antibodies with avidin-biotin conjugate rather than peroxidase-antiperoxidase) is used to identify tumor-associated antigens, viruses and other microorganisms, proteins, and hormones.

93. The answer is D. *(Anderson, 9/e. pp 1659–1661.)* Endometrial carcinoma affects menopausal and postmenopausal women, with the peak incidence at 55 to 65 years of age. Although it was much less common than squamous cervical cancer several decades ago, it has not been controlled as effectively as cervical cancer by the Papanicolaou smear technique and therapy, so that it is now more common than invasive cervical cancer. However, the major symptom of endometrial carcinoma, postmenopausal bleeding, results in diagnosis while the tumor is still confined to the uterus (stage I or II), which permits cure by surgery or radiotherapy. The annual death rate in the U.S. from endometrial cancer is 3000, while more than 6000 deaths result from squamous cervical cancer. Risk factors for endometrial cancer include obesity and glucose intolerance or diabetes.

94. The answer is E. *(Robbins, 4/e. pp 1355–1357.)* Diseases that lead to continued tissue synthesis and breakdown may produce hyperuricemia and clinical gout because of the resulting increase in nucleic acid turnover. This form of secondary gout may be seen in polycythemia vera, myeloid metaplasia, chronic leukemia, extensive psoriasis, and sarcoidosis. Cytotoxic drugs used in the chemotherapy of cancer may augment hyperuricemia. Decreased renal excretion of uric acid may also lead to secondary gout. Overproduction of uric acid may result from inborn errors of metabolism, as in the Lesch-Nyhan syndrome (deficiency of the enzyme hypoxanthine-guanine phosphoribosyltransferase (HGPRT.) Chondrocalcinosis is pseudogout.

95. The answer is A. *(Anderson, 9/e. pp 757–766.)* In atherosclerosis, primarily a disease of the arterial intima, disintegration of the internal elastic lamina is typical in advanced lesions, and necrosis commonly occurs at the base of the thickened intima. Essential lesions, occurring in the intima, are more numerous in larger than in smaller arteries. Although plaque formations cause little reduction in the size of the lumen of large arteries, atherosclerosis can lead to arterial dilatation and aneurysms. It is a progressive disease that begins early in life.

96. The answer is D. *(Robbins, 4/e. pp 1371–1373.)* Granular cell tumors (formerly known as *granular cell myoblastomas*) are benign neoplasms that frequently contain S-100 protein. They originate from Schwann-cell precursors. The most frequent locations are the tongue and subepidermal and subcutaneous tissues of the trunk (breast and many other sites). The eosinophilic cytoplasmic granules are phagolysosomes. These tumors are rarely malignant, though poorly encapsulated, and they frequently cause pseudoepitheliomatous hyperplasia of overlying epithelium, which is difficult to differentiate from squamous cell carcinoma.

97. The answer is E. *(Robbins, 4/e. pp 26, 950–953.)* *Hemochromatosis* is a generic term for disorders of iron overload marked by increases in total body iron and deposition of ferritin and hemosiderin in various organs with morphologic and functional damage to those organs. The pathogenesis is not fully understood but involves altered intestinal handling of iron with decreased postabsorption excretion, and alterations in iron metabolism and storage in reticuloendothelial cells. It causes a micronodular pigment cirrhosis with hemosiderin deposition in parenchymal, Kupffer, and bile duct epithelial cells, which is highlighted on Prussian blue staining. Hepatocellular carcinoma is a frequent (15 to 30 percent) complication of pigment cirrhosis. The pancreas shows intense pigmentation with atrophy and loss of parenchymal cells and diffuse interstitial fibrosis. Diabetes is a major feature of the clinical syndrome but is poorly correlated to the degree of iron deposition in the islets. Other tissues and organs that suffer major deposition of iron include the myocardium, the endocrine glands, skin (melanin and hemosiderin), and testes. Various tests useful in diagnosis reveal increased serum ferritin and plasma iron and decreased iron-binding capacity reflecting increased body iron load. Liver biopsy is definitive when it shows elevated hemosiderin content. Skin pigmentation is mainly due to increased amounts of melanin, seen with various types of cirrhosis.

98. The answer is D. (*Anderson, 9/e. pp 462, 467–468.*) Eggs of the roundworm *Ascaris* are found in contaminated soil in the southeastern United States. When swallowed, these eggs hatch, reach the small intestinal vessels, and travel to the lungs, where they may produce clinical bronchial asthma and pneumonitis. The New World hookworm, *Necator americanus,* penetrates exposed skin through exposure to larvae-containing soil; these infective filariform larvae reach the pulmonary circulation via the lymphatic and vascular systems and cause alveolar hemorrhages and temporary bronchopneumonia. Rhabditiform *Strongyloides* soil larvae also gain access to the vascular system and pulmonary circuit through penetration of exposed skin and also cause intraalveolar pneumonitis and hemorrhages. *Wuchereria bancrofti* filariae gain access to the human lymphatics (endolymphangitis, elephantiasis) via bites of the *Culex* mosquito; this organism is not noted for producing a pulmonary phase, but it does produce characteristic spermatic cord granulomas.

99. The answer is C. (*Robbins, 4/e. pp 61–62, 173–174, 696.*) The electron photomicrograph in the question shows a macrophage, the workhorse of the mononuclear phagocyte system. This wondrous cell is quite possibly the most active cell in the body. It certainly qualifies for the honor if multiple, varied functions are used to judge the competition. A partial list includes endocytosis (phagocytosis of particulate matter including injured cells and bacteria; pinocytosis of molecules in solution), antigen presentation and immunologic trafficking with sensitized T lymphocytes, and lysis of tumor cells. The macrophage also synthesizes and/or elaborates plasminogen activator, elastase, collagenase, some coagulation factors other than factor VIII (such as thromboplastin), neutrophilic chemotactic factor, mediators of inflammation, cyclooxygenase, lipoxygenase glycerol phosphocholine, components of complement, growth factors for wound healing, endogenous pyrogen (interleukin I), and probably other substances. Its internal machinery includes the work of acid hydrolytic enzymes in phagolysosomes. Mast cells and basophils degranulate in anaphylactic reactions. Factor VIII-vWF is a complex of coagulant (factor VIII, made in the liver) and von Willebrand's factor (vWF) that is synthesized in megakaryocytes and vascular endothelium.

100. The answer is B. *(Bullough, pp 2.2–2.6.)* Since the advent of the Jamshidi biopsy needle in the 1960s and proof that iliac crest marrow accurately reflects the state of the erythron, clinicians have not hesitated to perform or request bone marrow examinations of the iliac crest. The procedure's safety records are unquestioned. The practice of using bone marrow biopsy to define and document involvement of bone marrow by both solid and hematopoietic tumors has great value in the staging of patients. Similarly, documenting sideroblastic anemia by demonstrating the presence of ringed sideroblasts in the marrow has great value in clarifying anemias refractory to treatment. However, some clinicians injudiciously order bone marrow examinations in the investigation of iron deficiency anemia to identify stainable iron. In iron deficiency, the serum iron level is low, the iron-binding capacity is high, and the circulating serum transferrin level is high. After treatment with iron, the serum transferrin level will decrease. Nonmineralized bone (osteoid) covers most of the trabeculae and forms a substantial part of the bone tissue in osteomalacia. Determination of the amount of bone in the sample (e.g., the degree of osteopenia in metabolic bone disease) requires further histomorphometric analysis by computer.

101. The answer is E. *(Robbins, 4/e. pp 224–225, 233, 297–299.)* Immunodeficiency states often predispose to the development of neoplasia. The primary immunodeficiencies most clearly associated with an increased incidence of malignancy are common variable immunodeficiency, severe combined immunodeficiency, Wiskott-Aldrich syndrome, and ataxia-telangiectasia (in which defective repair of DNA may also play a role). The neoplasms in these genetic immunodeficiencies are predominantly non-Hodgkin's lymphomas, often immunoblastic, and often extranodal. Secondary immunodeficiency states occur in patients immunosuppressed for organ transplantation and tumors that develop are mainly high-grade, non-Hodgkin's lymphomas, frequently extranodal, especially in the CNS. Transplant patients also show an increased incidence of Kaposi's sarcoma, and a slight increase of squamous cell carcinoma in skin and oral tissues has been reported. The significant increase in neoplasia due to irradiation and radiomimetic drugs—primarily an increase in acute nonlymphoid leukemia—appears to be largely independent of immunosuppression. AIDS, a major devastating example of secondary immunodeficiency, was first recognized in 1981 through the increased incidence of Kaposi's sarcoma in young homosexual men. Subsequent studies established a considerable increase of high-grade, non-Hodgkin's lymphomas in patients infected with human immunodeficiency virus (HIV). Such lymphomas include small noncleaved cell, immunoblastic, and diffuse large cell lymphomas. There also may be an increase in Hodgkin's disease of aggressive type in HIV infection.

102. The answer is D. *(Henry, 18/e. p 1059. Morris, N Engl J Med 312:343, 1985.)* The *Vibrio* genus, including *V. cholerae,* is associated with gastrointestinal disease in the Far East, especially India, but is capable of inducing disease in the United States, as in pandemics occurring here around 1832 and in 1849. Along the coasts, especially the northeast and Gulf coasts of the United States, the vibrios increase in numbers in seawater and in seafood and are more likely to cause infections during the late summer and early autumn months. Patients with underlying liver disease, such as alcoholics, and those with immunosuppressive disorders are advised not to ingest raw shellfish during these months because of an increased incidence of disease with the vibrio organisms in these patients. The mycobacteria are acid-fast bacilli associated with tuberculosis and tuberculosis-like diseases; *M. avium-intracellulare* is known to be a frequent organism in AIDS. These organisms are not curved as the vibrios are.

103. The answer is D. *(Robbins, 4/e. pp 56–57.)* Leukocytes, including basophils, are involved with the production of derivatives of a very important polyunsaturated fatty acid, arachidonic acid. By a complex two-path cascade system, the metabolites of arachidonic acid eventually yield prostaglandins (vasodilators) and leukotrienes (vasoconstrictors). The biosynthesis begins by activation of cell phospholipase A_2 and C and proceeds either by the action of fatty acid cyclooxygenase on arachidonic acid to form prostaglandins, or by the action of lipoxygenase to yield leukotrienes (hydroperoxyeicosatetraenoic acid in platelets, mast cells, and leukocytes). While many substances can be chemotactic, few are known to be as potent as several of the leukotrienes. Leukotriene B_4 as a chemotactic agent is involved in neutrophil aggregation, while leukotrienes TC_4, TD_4, and TE_4 are involved with increased vascular permeability, bronchoconstriction, and vasoconstriction. Prostaglandin E and prostacyclin probably account for most vasodilatation seen in inflammation. Thus both leukotrienes and prostaglandins contribute to edema. Leukotrienes C_4, D_4, and E_4 are extremely potent in increasing vascular permeability, as is platelet activating factor.

104. The answer is A. *(Robbins, 4/e. pp 1192–1193.)* Long and continuous exposure to endogenous estrogens increases the risk of developing breast carcinoma. Therefore, late menopause (after age 50), early menarche (especially before age 13), and nulliparity are all risk factors. Endometrial adenocarcinoma and occasional ovarian cancers are also associated with continuous estrogen stimulation with a resultant higher risk of the development of breast cancer in the same patient. Other factors include Jewish ancestry and obesity—estrogen metabolism is altered in obese women and synthesis of estrone increased. Family history is significant, especially if mother and sister had premenopausal breast cancer, in which case there is an increased risk of 50 times that of controls. A past history of breast cancer, especially of lobular type, means greater risk of contralateral breast carcinoma. Hormonal and genetic factors and obesity are probably the major risk factors.

105–107. The answers are: 105-B, 106-E, 107-C. *(Robbins, 4/e. pp 137, 145–147, 154, 626, 777, 1356–1357.)* Fabry's disease, seen mostly in males, is characterized by accumulation of glycosphingolipid (trihexosylceramide) in the cardiovascular-renal system, skin, and eyes due to a deficiency of α-galactosidase A. Angiokeratomas of the skin (small, red, raised lesions) usually appear in childhood and increase with age, often in a "swim suit" distribution on buttocks, back, genitalia, and inner thighs. Burning pain in hands and feet, triggered by exercise or stress, and diminished ability to sweat are common. Ocular abnormalities—tortuous conjunctival vessels and corneal opacity—are suggestive. Inheritance is X-linked recessive and female carriers develop angiokeratomas, eye changes, and burning pains, without the renal and cardiac problems of males. Renal dialysis and transplantation have now improved prognosis. Prenatal diagnosis is done by amniocentesis or chorionic villus sampling and the disorder occurs in about one in 40,000 persons.

Tay-Sachs disease (TSD), or G_{M2} gangliosidosis type I, is a storage disease in which this ganglioside accumulates in neurons of the central and autonomic nervous systems and retina because of deficient hexosaminidase A. Inherited as an autosomal recessive trait, TSD is found primarily but not exclusively among Ashkenazi Jews and among a group of non-Jewish French Canadians. Thousands of carriers of the TSD gene have been identified, and prenatal diagnosis is possible by assay for hexosaminidase A activity in cultured fetal cells. Major clinical features include mental-motor deterioration, blindness, a cherry-red spot in the macula, and death by three years of age.

The fragile X syndrome, transmitted as an X-linked recessive trait, is the second most common cause of genetic mental retardation after Down's syndrome. The cytogenetic abnormality of discontinuous staining or secondary constriction (fragile region) occurs at the end of the long arm of the X chromosome (Xq 27.3). Major characteristics include mental retardation and macroorchidism. Fragile X syndrome is not a typical X-linked trait since 20 percent of fragile X males are symptomless carriers who can pass the abnormal chromosome to their daughters, while one-third of female carriers exhibit some symptoms. The syndrome is probably responsible for 10 percent of mentally retarded males.

108–111. The answers are: 108-A, 109-B, 110-D, 111-C. *(Robbins, 4/e. pp 441, 449–452, 454–459.)* Pyridoxine deficiency should be rare but is fairly common because of drugs that act as pyridoxine antagonists. Pyridoxal phosphate is important for numerous enzyme reactions in amino acid metabolism, in heme synthesis, and for normal neuronal excitability. Peripheral neuritis, seizures, microcytic anemia, and often dermatitis and glossitis suggest the deficiency. Many drugs may act as antagonists of vitamin B_6: estrogens inhibit its role in tryptophan metabolism, isoniazid can inhibit enzymes that use pyridoxine as a cofactor (thus inducing seizures), and penicillamine acts in the same way. A common cause of B_6 deficiency is chronic alcoholism.

Ascorbic acid, a redox agent, is essential in collagen synthesis, so deficiency in vitamin C means defective collagen synthesis resulting in fragile capillaries and hemorrhagic areas around hair follicles, abnormal hair development, splinter hemorrhages in the nail beds, and hematomas. The syndrome is common in elderly people living on a diet deficient in milk, fruits, and vegetables.

Folate deficiency may be present with scurvy and causes a macrocytic anemia similar to the megaloblastic anemia of vitamin B_{12} deficiency, but without gastric atrophy or neurologic changes. Deficiency occurs in chronic alcoholics, the elderly, and malabsorption syndromes (sprue) or with folate antagonists (methotrexate) used in cancer chemotherapy.

Thiamine deficiency occurs in alcoholics and prisoners of war because of poor diet, deficient absorption and storage, and accelerated destruction of thiamine diphosphate. Major manifestations are both cardiovascular, with tachycardia an early sign of peripheral vasodilatation, and neurologic, with resultant beriberi. Nystagmus, ataxia, and confusion—often with bilateral lateral rectus, or 6th nerve, palsies (ophthalmoplegia)—indicate Wernicke's encephalopathy. The lack of B_1 has caused damage to areas of thalamus, hypothalamus, midbrain, and cerebellar vermis. The classic triad of confusion, ataxia, and ophthalmoplegia is not common and some patients remain undiagnosed. Others who recover after thiamine administration from the acute encephalopathy are left with major defects in retrograde memory and learning (Korsakoff syndrome).

Night blindness is the earliest symptom of vitamin A deficiency, followed by conjunctival changes—xerophthalmia (dry cornea and conjunctiva) and keratomalacia. Deficiency also leads to squamous metaplasia in trachea and bronchi, and such metaplasia in sebaceous and sweat glands of dry skin causes follicular hyperkeratosis and predisposes to acne.

112–115. The answers are: 112-B , 113-C, 114-A, 115-D. *(Robbins, 4/e. pp 325, 332, 335, 386–387, 390–391, 394–396.)* *Histoplasma capsulatum* causes one of the three major fungal infections in the United States that may result in systemic infection (*Blastomyces* and *Coccidioides* are the other two). Although it commonly produces asymptomatic primary disease, it can result in striking granulomatous inflammation with granulomatous lung disease and possibly sclerosing mediastinitis. Seen most frequently in the Midwest and inhaled from contaminated soil, it forms a yeastlike pathogenic phase in the host and may cause acute, chronic progressive, or asymptomatic disease, the last being the most common outcome.

Cryptococcal infection is the most common fungal CNS infection in the immunocompromised, especially in persons with AIDS or leukemia, lymphoma, and Hodgkin's disease. The soil-dwelling yeast is inhaled, but lung involvement is mild, at least in the nonimmunodeficient. Diagnosis of the dangerous cryptococcal meningitis is achieved by finding encapsulated yeasts in CSF preparations treated with India ink to expose the wide capsules by negative staining (positive in only 50 percent of cases in which diagnosis is eventually made). The CSF and serum should be tested for cryptococcal antigen by the latex cryptococcal agglutination test (LCAT), which is positive in more than 90 percent of cases. Cryptococcal meningitis varies from a chronic inflammatory and granulomatous infection to a noninflammatory meningitis with numerous yeasts massed, sometimes forming cystic "soap-bubble" lesions in the brain.

Rocky Mountain spotted fever is transmitted to man by ticks, as is Lyme disease. Rocky Mountain spotted fever—an acute infectious disease caused by *Rickettsia rickettsii* and characterized by muscle pain, high fever, and skin eruptions—is endemic throughout North America, Rickettsiae typically invade the walls of blood vessels with resultant hemorrhage and thrombosis.

Yellow fever is an acute infectious disease of variable severity and short duration. It is an arthropod-borne (*Aedes* mosquito), hemorrhagic disease of subtropical and tropical New World areas, caused by a single-stranded RNA togavirus. It results in hepatocellular damage with jaundice and hematemesis.

Gram-negative bacteria have cell walls containing endotoxins (lipopolysaccharide-protein complexes) that are released from disintegrating bacteria to cause such effects of gram-negative sepsis as fever, increased capillary permeability with shock, and disseminated intravascular coagulation.

116–119. The answers are: 116-C, 117-D, 118-E, 119-B. *(Robbins, 4/e. pp 1453, 1454, 1460, 1461.)* Long-standing diabetes mellitus is a major cause of blindness in the United States and Europe (25 percent of cases of acquired blindness in the U.S.). Diabetic retinopathy is the most common form, but cataracts and glaucoma occur also. Two major types of diabetic retinopathy, nonproliferative and proliferative, exist with the former characterized by microaneurysms, hemorrhages, and thickened retinal capillaries (microangiopathy). In proliferative retinopathy, new capillary formation and fibrosis eventually lead to blindness or decreased visual acuity.

Keratomalacia, which is due to severe, protracted vitamin A deficiency, is a major problem in Southeast Asia, Africa, and Central and South America, where it causes blindness in about one quarter million children annually. Dryness, softening, and destruction of the cornea occur, while characteristic eye changes include Bitot's spots—a localized form of keratomalacia with small gray plaques representing thickened, keratinized epithelium.

Trachoma, a common cause of blindness in hot, arid regions of the Third World, is caused by *Chlamydia trachomatis,* serotypes A to C. Conjunctival infection is followed by lymphoid follicular hyperplasia and, subsequently, pannus invades the cornea and leads to blindness.

Retinitis pigmentosa is a rare degeneration of the retinal outer receptor layer and underlying pigment epithelium; it is inherited as an autosomal dominant, or recessive, or sex-linked recessive trait. Losses of night vision and, eventually, central vision are prominent.

Silver-wire arterioles are seen in severe arteriosclerotic retinopathy when sclerotic opacity obscures intravascular blood completely.

120–123. The answers are: 120-C, 121-E, 122-A, 123-D. *(Robbins, 4/e. pp 173–180, 743–744, 1040–1041, 1044.)* All five immunoglobulins are polypeptides with two light and two heavy chains linked by disulfide bonds. The Ig molecule consists of two fragments of Fab, which are capable of binding antigen, and one Fc fragment. Light chains are two types, kappa and lambda. Heavy chains are of five major types forming five distinct immunoglobulin classes on the basis of the heavy chains that account for the antigenic differences.

IgA is synthesized by mucosal plasma cells of the GI tract, lung, and urinary tract—thus making it the immunoglobulin of "secretory immunity"—and is found in saliva, sweat, nasal secretion, and tears. It is secreted as dimer bound to a secretory piece that stabilizes the molecule against proteolysis. In IgA nephropathy (Berger's disease), circulating IgA immune complex is present in 50 percent of patients and a diffuse renal mesangial proliferation with IgA deposition occurs.

Local anaphylactic reactions include hay fever, bronchial asthma, certain food allergies, and urticarial reactions to drugs or injected antigens. Systemic anaphylaxis may result from injection of antisera or penicillin and may cause severe shock or death. Type I hypersensitivity (anaphylaxis) occurs when exposure to antigen leads to production of cytotropic IgE antibodies that become fixed by their Fc portions to mast cells and basophils. On reexposure, antigen combines with the cell-bound antibody and this is followed by mast cell degranulation with discharge of primary mediators (histamine). Secondary mediators (leukotrienes, prostaglandin) are released via cell membrane phospholipids.

IgM is the first immunoglobulin to respond to an antigenic stimulus and is the largest Ig. Waldenström's macroglobulinemia is a plasma cell dyscrasia characterized by infiltration of bone marrow, lymph nodes, liver, and spleen by neoplastic B cells that secrete a monoclonal IgM immunoglobulin, leading to macroglobulinemia. Serum electrophoresis shows an M-protein spike and diagnosis rests on the typical bone marrow findings and the M-protein spike due to IgM in the serum.

Most of the circulating human gamma globulin (80 percent) is of the IgG class. It crosses the placenta and is the major protective immunoglobulin in the neonate. IgG has Fc receptors and activates complement.

Hematology

DIRECTIONS: Each question below contains five suggested responses. Select the **one best** response to each question.

124. The photomicrograph below was taken from a soft tissue swelling in the cheek and mandible of a 17-year-old female patient. The cytoplasmic vacuoles would react with which one of the following?

(A) Myeloperoxidase
(B) Oil red O
(C) Nonspecific esterase
(D) Chloracetate esterase
(E) Periodic acid–Schiff (PAS)

125. The neutrophil in the photomicrograph shown below was obtained from peripheral blood and is most likely to be found in association with

(A) folic acid deficiency
(B) infection
(C) iron deficiency
(D) malignancy
(E) ingestion of a marrow-toxic agent

126. The graph below depicts the results of a red cell osmotic fragility test. The broken-line curve represents which of the following?

(A) Glucose-6-phosphate dehydrogenase deficiency
(B) Thalassemia
(C) Hereditary spherocytosis
(D) Drug-induced hemolytic anemia
(E) Normal response

127. In the photomicrograph below, the nucleated cell that is located next to the neutrophil has a gray-pink cytoplasm and is

(A) a polychromatophilic megaloblast
(B) a plasma cell
(C) an orthochromatic normoblast
(D) a myelocyte
(E) a myeloblast

---

128. Which of the following laboratory findings is LEAST likely to be present in a patient with sickle cell anemia?

(A) Normochromic anemia
(B) Increased number of target cells
(C) Elevated reticulocyte count
(D) Elevated erythrocyte sedimentation rate
(E) Increased hemoglobin F

129. True statements regarding nodular sclerosing Hodgkin's disease include that it

(A) is more common in males
(B) usually affects elderly people
(C) is characterized by the presence of lacunar cells
(D) commonly affects Waldeyer's ring
(E) usually involves infradiaphragmatic lymph nodes

130. The causes of secondary aplastic anemia include all the following EXCEPT

(A) whole body irradiation
(B) alkylating agents
(C) chloramphenicol
(D) myelophthisic anemia
(E) viral hepatitis

131. Vitamin K is required for the synthesis of all the following EXCEPT

(A) prothrombin
(B) clotting factor VII
(C) clotting factor VIII
(D) clotting factor IX
(E) clotting factor X

132. The photomicrograph below is of peripheral blood from a patient with splenomegaly, anemia, and pancytopenia. If hairy cell leukemia is suspected, which of the following would be useful in establishing the diagnosis?

(A) Myeloperoxidase stain
(B) Sudan black B
(C) Acid phosphatase stain
(D) Leukocyte alkaline phosphatase
(E) Nonspecific esterase

133. Which of the following substances inhibits platelet aggregation?

(A) Prostacyclin (PGI$_2$)
(B) Epinephrine
(C) Adenosine diphosphate
(D) 5-Hydroxytryptamine
(E) Thrombin

134. Acute idiopathic thrombocytopenic purpura (ITP) in children is characterized by

(A) an insidious onset
(B) being more common in females
(C) a history of recent viral infection
(D) megakaryocytic hypoplasia
(E) a high mortality

135. The photomicrograph below is of the spleen from an adult patient who had marked splenomegaly. Which of the following abnormalities is most compatible with the changes seen in the spleen?

(A) Reduced levels of glucocerebrosidase activity
(B) Glucose-6-phosphate dehydrogenase deficiency
(C) Glucuronidase deficiency
(D) Lysosomal glucosidase deficiency
(E) Trihexosylceramide α-galactosidase deficiency

136. An 11-year-old Jamaican boy develops a massive benign enlargement of the cervical lymph nodes associated with fever and leukocytosis. Which of the following lymph node disorders could account for these findings?

(A) Toxoplasmosis
(B) Histiocytic medullary reticulosis
(C) Burkitt's disease
(D) Sinus histiocytosis with massive lymphadenopathy (SHML)
(E) Angioimmunoblastic lymphadenopathy with dysproteinemia

137. The photomicrograph below was taken after 30 min of incubation at 37°C of a mixture of one drop of blood and two drops of an aqueous 2% sodium metabisulfite solution. The appearance of the erythrocytes in this preparation shows that they contain

(A) hemoglobin A
(B) hemoglobin A$_2$
(C) hemoglobin C
(D) hemoglobin F
(E) hemoglobin S

138. The photomicrograph below is from the bone marrow of a patient with weakness. All the following may be associated with this abnormality EXCEPT

(A) pernicious anemia
(B) hyperthyroidism
(C) celiac disease
(D) HTLV
(E) alcoholism

139. The cells shown in the photomicrograph below are usually increased in the peripheral blood in all the following EXCEPT

(A) eczema and pemphigus
(B) bronchial asthma
(C) some cases of Hodgkin's disease
(D) adrenocortical stimulation
(E) parasitic infections

140. Typical findings in a patient with von Willebrand's disease include all the following EXCEPT

(A) decreased levels of factor VIII
(B) decreased glass bead adhesion of platelets
(C) prolonged bleeding time
(D) frequent hemarthrosis and spontaneous joint hemorrhage
(E) menorrhagia

141. δ-Aminolevulinic acid is excreted in increased amounts in the urine of patients with

(A) lead poisoning
(B) carcinoma of the pancreas
(C) chronic pyelonephritis
(D) vitamin C intoxication
(E) ulcerative colitis

142. A bone marrow aspirate was obtained from a 70-year-old man whose symptoms included weakness, weight loss, and recurrent infections. Laboratory findings included proteinuria, anemia, and an abnormal component in serum proteins. A photomicrograph of the bone marrow aspirate is shown below. The most probable diagnosis is

(A) monomyelocytic leukemia
(B) histiocytic leukemia
(C) multiple myeloma
(D) Gaucher's disease
(E) leukemic reticuloendotheliosis

Questions 143–144

143. The cell in the photomicrograph above was found in a bone
marrow aspirate from a 25-year-old
man. Such a cell is generally considered pathognomonic for

(A) Niemann-Pick disease
(B) histiocytic lymphoma
(C) megaloblastic anemia
(D) Gaucher's disease
(E) myelogenous leukemia

144. All the following statements
concerning the disease associated
with the cell shown above are true
EXCEPT

(A) the pathognomonic cells are
typically 20 to 100 μm in diameter and have a wrinkled, striated
cytoplasm
(B) inheritance is autosomal dominant with variable penetrance
(C) the serum level of acid phosphatase is frequently elevated
(D) an excess amount of sphingo-
lipid is stored in body tissues
(E) three types of the disease can be
differentiated genetically and
clinically

145. A woman who is 5 weeks post partum (normal delivery, healthy child) develops bleeding episodes with oliguria and hematuria. No fever or neuro-logic manifestations are present. The blood urea nitrogen level is 65 mg/dL; a peripheral blood smear is presented in the photomicrograph below. This patient most likely has

(A) thrombotic thrombocytopenic purpura
(B) autoimmune thrombocytopenic purpura
(C) hemolytic uremic syndrome
(D) disseminated intravascular coagulopathy
(E) sickle cell crisis

146. All the following are known to cause splenomegaly EXCEPT

(A) sickle cell disease
(B) Hodgkin's disease
(C) chronic lymphocytic leukemia (CLL)
(D) hairy cell leukemia
(E) polycythemia vera

147. Non-Hodgkin's lymphomas (NHLs) that exhibit a nodular growth pattern may be character-ized by which of the following?

(A) Increased frequency in adoles-cents
(B) Predominant T cell type
(C) Better prognosis than in the dif-fuse type
(D) Predominance in males
(E) Well-differentiated lymphocytic lymphoma

148. A 38-year-old man presents with a red, maculopapular rash, Coombs-positive hemolytic anemia, generalized lymphadenopathy, splenomegaly, hepatomegaly, fever, fatigue, and weight loss. The lymph node biopsy specimen seen in the photomicrograph below shows effacement and vascular proliferation. This constellation points to a diagnosis of

(A) lymphopathia venereum
(B) immunoblastic lymphadenopathy
(C) mucocutaneous lymph node syndrome
(D) acute leukemia
(E) malignant histiocytosis

149. The presence in serum of a mu heavy-chain protein is a distinctive feature of which of the following diseases?

(A) Chronic lymphocytic leukemia
(B) Macroglobulinemia
(C) Lymphocytic lymphoma
(D) Plasma cell myeloma
(E) Multiple myeloma

150. A 20-year-old man presents in the emergency room with a lymphoma involving the mediastinum that is producing respiratory distress. The lymphocytes are most likely to have cell surface markers characteristic of which of the following?

(A) B cells
(B) T cells
(C) Macrophages
(D) Dendritic reticulum cells
(E) Langerhans cells

151. The cells seen in the photomicrograph below were removed from an anemic patient and stained with an iron stain. This patient is most likely to have

(A) iron deficiency anemia
(B) acute blood loss
(C) B_{12} deficiency
(D) B_2 deficiency
(E) pyridoxine deficiency

152. Transferrin shows all the following characteristics EXCEPT

(A) normally about 33 percent saturation with iron
(B) increased saturation in hemochromatosis
(C) increased saturation in severe liver disease
(D) decreased saturation in marrow hypoplasia
(E) decreased saturation in iron deficiency anemia

153. An anemic patient has the following red cell indexes: mean corpuscular volume, 70 μm^3 (normal: 90 ± 7); mean corpuscular hemoglobin, 22 g/dL (normal: 29 ± 2); and mean corpuscular hemoglobin concentration, 34 percent (normal: 34 ± 2). These values are most consistent with a diagnosis of

(A) folic acid deficiency anemia
(B) iron deficiency anemia
(C) pernicious anemia
(D) thalassemia minor
(E) sideroblastic anemia

154. The bone marrow biopsy shown below was performed because of splenomegaly and anemia in an adult. On the basis of the appearance of the bone marrow core, choose the most likely diagnosis.

(A) Chronic myeloid leukemia (CML)
(B) Aplastic anemia
(C) Acute leukemia
(D) Myeloid metaplasia with myelofibrosis
(E) Microangiopathic hemolytic anemia

155. Chronic myeloid leukemia is LEAST likely to be associated with

(A) splenomegaly
(B) basophilia
(C) translocation t (8;14)
(D) thrombocytosis
(E) low leukocyte alkaline phosphatase

156. During the induction of an immune response, which cell is thought to process the initiating antigen?

(A) Eosinophil
(B) Basophil
(C) Macrophage
(D) T cell
(E) B cell

157. An elderly woman enters the hospital with an abdominal mass, anemia, and weakness. At surgery, an infiltrating retroperitoneal mass is found involving the mesenteric lymph nodes and right kidney. A biopsy specimen from one of the lymph nodes is shown and is compatible with large-cell immunoblastic lymphoma. This neoplasm is associated with all the following EXCEPT

(A) predominant B-cell origin
(B) prior immunologic disorder
(C) early dissemination to bone marrow
(D) rapid death if untreated
(E) plasmacytoid or polymorphous features

158. A young child has recurrent bacterial infections, eczema, thrombocytopenia, lymphadenopathy, and the absence of delayed-type hypersensitivity. The most likely diagnosis is

(A) Pelger-Huët anomaly
(B) Wiskott-Aldrich syndrome
(C) Chédiak-Higashi syndrome
(D) chronic granulomatous disease of childhood
(E) nodular-sclerosing Hodgkin's disease

159. A 25-year-old woman with known systemic lupus erythematosus presents with jaundice, splenomegaly, peripheral blood schistocytes, and a reticulocyte count of 24 percent. The antibody most likely to be responsible for this complex reacts in vitro at

(A) 5°C
(B) 20°C
(C) 25°C
(D) 37°C
(E) 56°C

160. The binucleate or bilobed giant cell with prominent acidophilic "owl-eye" nucleoli shown in the photomicrograph below is correctly characterized by which of the following statements?

(A) It is diagnostic of cytomegalic inclusion disease
(B) It is sometimes referred to as the lacunar cell
(C) It is necessary but not sufficient for the diagnosis of Hodgkin's disease
(D) It is a rapidly proliferating tumor cell seen in middivision
(E) None of the above

161. A 19-year-old man presents with a sore throat, malaise, and cervical lymphadenopathy. Peripheral blood film shows lymphocytosis with many lymphocytes that show atypical nuclei and abundant basophilic cytoplasm. The most appropriate course of action is

(A) lymph node biopsy
(B) bone marrow biopsy
(C) prompt treatment with ampicillin
(D) heterophil test
(E) serum IgM anti-EBV

162. In polycythemia rubra vera (PRV),

(A) the bone marrow shows selective erythroid hyperplasia
(B) hemorrhagic phenomena are uncommon
(C) the spleen is usually markedly enlarged
(D) the platelet count is typically <150,000/mm^3
(E) leukocyte alkaline phosphate levels are elevated

DIRECTIONS: The groups of questions below consist of lettered headings followed by a set of numbered items. For each numbered item select the **one** lettered heading with which it is **most** closely associated. Each lettered heading may be used **once, more than once, or not at all.**

Questions 163–167

For each description below, choose the type of leukemia with which it is most likely to be associated.

(A) Acute lymphoblastic leukemia
(B) Acute myeloblastic leukemia (M1)
(C) Acute promyelocytic leukemia (M3)
(D) Chronic lymphocytic leukemia
(E) Hairy cell leukemia

163. Auer rods are frequently present in the leukemic cells

164. It is associated with a short course and diffuse intravascular coagulation

165. It occurs in older adults, produces relatively few symptoms, and is associated with the longest survival

166. The enzyme TdT is often present in leukemic cells; lymphadenopathy is characteristic and striking

167. It constitutes about 20 percent of childhood leukemias and relapse is common following chemotherapy in older adults

Questions 168–170

For each disease listed below, choose the appropriate chromosomal translocation and associated oncogene.

(A) t8;14, c-*myc*
(B) t8;21, c-*mos*
(C) t9;22, c-*abl*
(D) t15;17, c-*fes*
(E) t14;18, *bcl*-2

168. Follicular lymphoma

169. Chronic myeloid leukemia

170. Burkitt's lymphoma

Questions 171–174

For each of the proteins listed, choose the disease with which it is most likely to be associated.

(A) Rheumatoid arthritis
(B) Senile cardiac amyloidosis
(C) Nodular lymphoma
(D) Alzheimer's disease
(E) Medullary carcinoma of the thyroid

171. Amyloid light chain (AL) protein

172. Amyloid-associated (AA) protein

173. Beta$_2$ amyloid protein

174. Transthyretin

Hematology

Answers

124. The answer is B. *(Henry, 18/e. pp 701, 710–711. Robbins, 4/e. pp 715–716.)* Burkitt's lymphoma, or undifferentiated lymphoma, is characterized by a rapid proliferation of primitive lymphoid cells with thick nuclear membranes, multiple nucleoli, and intensely basophilic cytoplasm when stained with Wright's stain. The cells are often mixed with macrophages in biopsy, giving a starry-sky appearance. The vacuoles contain lipid and this would be reflected by a positive oil-red-O reaction. PAS stain is nonspecific but does mark neutrophils and acute lymphoblastic leukemia cells. Nonspecific esterase is found predominantly within monocytes but also in megakaryocytes and to a minor extent in myelomonocytes. Chloracetate esterase and myeloperoxidase are primarily found within the lysosomes of granulocytes, including neutrophils, promyelocytes, and faintly in rare monocytes.

125. The answer is A. *(Robbins, 4/e. pp 679–685.)* In contrast to a normal, mature neutrophil, which has from two to five nuclear lobes, the neutrophil shown has at least six lobes and is an illustration of neutrophilic hypersegmentation. Granulocytic hypersegmentation is significant and among the first hematologic findings in the peripheral blood of patients who have megaloblastic anemia in its developmental stages. Neutrophilic hypersegmentation is generally considered a sensitive indicator of megaloblastic anemia, which can be caused by a deficiency either in vitamin B_{12}, in folate, or in both.

126. The answer is C. *(Henry, 18/e. pp 644–645. Robbins, 4/e. pp 663–665.)* Spherocytes in a peripheral blood smear show a smaller diameter than normal and an apparent increase in hemoglobin concentration because of a decrease in cell surface, with consequent deeper staining for hemoglobin. Spectrin lacks the ability to bind protein 4.1 in this autosomal dominant disorder, yielding a skeleton defect of the red cell membrane. Other proteins that help maintain the shape of the red cell include protein 3 and ankyrin, which bridges the spectrin and the cell membrane protein 3. The disorder can be diagnosed in the laboratory by the osmotic fragility test (which the graph shows, with the shaded area reflecting a normal response to a hypotonic solution). Spherocytes will lyse at a higher concentration of sodium chloride than will normal red cells. Flat hypochromic cells, as those in thalassemia, have a greater capacity to expand in dilute salt solution and thus lyse at a lower concentration (which is seen in the unbroken curve to the far right). The longer the incubation of the red cells in these salt concentrations, the greater the response to osmotic change.

127. The answer is A. *(Williams, 4/e. pp 453–454.)* The cell in question is much larger than the other red cells and has an immature nucleus with coarse, clumped chromatin. These features help to identify it as a nucleated red cell exhibiting megaloblastic maturation. The cell might be confused with a plasma cell, but plasma cells exhibit clumped chromatin that stains a dark purple, a deep blue cytoplasm, and nuclei that are small and eccentric and often lie next to perinuclear clear zones.

128. The answer is D. *(Wilson, 12/e. pp 1544–1547.)* Blood from patients who have sickle cell anemia exhibits a low erythrocyte sedimentation rate (ESR). The irregular shape of sickle cells prevents the rouleaux formation that is prerequisite for a normal ESR. Sickle cell anemia is classified as a normocytic, normochromic, and hemolytic anemia in which target cells, found in increased numbers, can compose up to 30 percent of peripheral blood cells, and in which reticulocytosis—as a reflection of an increased rate of erythropoiesis in the hyperplastic bone marrow—is persistently 10 percent above normal. In addition, electrophoretic findings reveal an elevation of hemoglobin F up to 40 percent, the presence of hemoglobin S in a range of 60 to 99 percent, and the absence of hemoglobin A.

129. The answer is C. *(Robbins, 4/e. pp 717–722.)* Hodgkin's disease is broadly divided into four histologic subtypes, the most common of which is the nodular sclerosis variant. This is characterized morphologically by the presence of the lacunar variant of Reed-Sternberg cells and by bands of fibrous tissue that divide the lymph node into nodules. Unlike the other subtypes of Hodgkin's disease, it is more common in females. Young adults are classically affected and the disease typically involves the cervical, supraclavicular, or mediastinal lymph nodes. Involvement of extranodal lymphoid tissue is unusual.

130. The answer is D. *(Robbins, 4/e. pp 688–690.)* Hematopoietic stem cell failure occurs in aplastic anemia, probably because of defective stem cells or their immunologic suppression. Pancytopenia results, although selective suppression with pure red cell aplasia, agranulocytosis, or thrombocytopenia may occur. In 50 percent of cases, aplastic anemia is idiopathic or primary, but there are many physical and chemical causes of secondary aplastic anemia. Whole body irradiation is the major physical cause. Chemical causes include many drugs, such as alkylating agents, antimetabolites, and the antibiotic chloramphenicol. Severe aplastic anemia may occur following viral hepatitis of the non-A, non-B type, or following infectious mononucleosis. In myelophthisic anemia, marrow failure is due to marrow replacement by metastatic tumor or other lesions, but no association with stem cell defects exists.

131. The answer is C. *(Williams, 4/e. pp 1285–1286.)* Vitamin K is not required for the biosynthesis of coagulation factor VIII, which has an uncertain participation as a trace protein in the intrinsic coagulation pathway and is also known as the antihemophilic factor. Vitamin K, although its biochemical mode of action remains unclear, is required for the biosynthesis and maintenance of normal concentrations of coagulation factors II (prothrombin), VII, IX, and X.

132. The answer is C. *(Williams, 4/e. pp 1025–1028.)* Since 1966, hairy cell leukemia has been diagnosed with increasing frequency. This specialized form of leukemia should be suspected in patients with splenomegaly; pancytopenia, including thrombocytopenia; bleeding; fatigue; and leukemic lymphocyte-like cells in the peripheral blood demonstrating cytoplasmic projections at the cell periphery ("hairy" cells). These cells stain for acid phosphatase, and the reaction is refractory to treatment with tartaric acid (tartrate-resistant acid phosphatase, or TRAP).

133. The answer is A. *(Robbins, 4/e. pp 95–97.)* Prostacyclin inhibits platelet aggregation, probably by increasing cyclic AMP levels within the platelets, whereas all the other agents listed promote it. Other potent inhibitors of platelet aggregation include mercurials and chemicals that react with sulfhydryl groups.

134. The answer is C. *(Robbins, 4/e. pp 692–695.)* In acute idiopathic thrombocytopenic purpura (ITP), which occurs predominantly in children under 8 years of age, there is an acute onset about 2 weeks after a viral infection (rubella, viral hepatitis, infectious mononucleosis). There is no female predominance as seen in chronic ITP, which is most frequent in women 20 to 50 years old and is characterized by an insidious onset. Both acute and chronic forms are associated with increased platelet destruction and normal or increased megakaryocytes in bone marrow. Most patients with acute ITP make a spontaneous recovery, although cerebral hemorrhage may occur and accounts for most of the few deaths.

135. The answer is A. *(Robbins, 4/e. pp 146–154.)* The photomicrograph in the question shows the presence of lipid-laden macrophages replacing much of the splenic parenchyma. The macrophages have a somewhat vacuolated cytoplasm, which is characteristic of Gaucher's disease. This is an autosomal recessive disease characterized by a reduction or a deficiency of glucocerebrosidase. Thus glucocerebroside accumulates mainly in the mononuclear phagocytic system. Three clinical types occur. The classic is type I, which occurs in adults and generally spares the central nervous system with the glucocerebrosides limited to the mononuclear phagocyte system of the spleen, liver, and bone marrow. This is mainly found in European Jewish patients and is the most common form of Gaucher's disease. Type II is the infantile form, which involves the brain and presents no detectable glucocerebrosidase activity. Death occurs at an early age. Type III may be thought of as being an intermediate between types I and II; it is found in adolescent patients and mainly involves the mononuclear phagocyte system early but will involve the brain by the third decade of life. Trihexosylceramide α-galactosidase deficiency is Fabry's disease, which is characterized by angiokeratomas of the skin resulting in marked ceramide trihexoside accumulations within the endothelial and smooth muscle cells of blood vessels, ganglion cells, heart, renal tubules, and glomeruli. Glucosidase deficiency is type II glycogen storage disease, which is one of the variants of liver phosphorylase deficiency. Glucose-6-phosphate dehydrogenase deficiency results in hemolytic disease in both sexes, with the male more severely affected.

136. The answer is D. *(Anderson, 9/e. pp 1436, 1440–1442.)* Clinicians and pathologists alike should be familiar with the benign syndrome of lymph node enlargement called *sinus histiocytosis with massive lymphadenopathy*. This is a self-limiting, invariably benign disorder found classically in young, black, African and Caribbean patients, but it has been found in others as well. It is characterized clinically by profound enlargement of regional cervical lymph nodes, fever, and leukocytosis. Histologically, the lymph nodes show marked histiocytic proliferation within the sinuses, with engulfment of lymphocytes within the histiocytes. There may be skin involvement, and histiocytes containing phagocytosed lymphocytes may be present in the skin biopsy specimen. The patients predictably revert to normal within a period of months. Histiocytic medullary reticulosis is a disease in which a form of malignant histiocytes is found in lymph node sinuses, with engulfed red cells found within the neoplastic histiocytes (erythrophagocytosis). Primitive, round lymphoblastic tumor cells are found in tissue taken from patients with Burkitt's lymphoma.

137. The answer is E. *(Henry, 18/e. p 652.)* The photomicrograph shown in the question demonstrates the results of the metabisulfite sickling test for detecting the presence of hemoglobin S. The test does not differentiate homozygous from heterozygous states. Red cells that contain large amounts of normal or abnormal hemoglobins other than S rarely exhibit sickling. The test is based on the fact that erythrocytes containing a large proportion of hemoglobin S sickle in solutions of low oxygen content. Metabisulfite is a reducing substance that enhances the process of deoxygenation.

138. The answer is D. *(Robbins, 4/e. pp 679–685.)* The photomicrograph in the question shows the presence of megaloblasts accompanied by unusually large neutrophils and precursors. These abnormalities may be caused by either a deficiency or lack of absorption of vitamin B_{12} or of folic acid. In addition to diets deficient in these two substances, any condition leading to poor absorption of them will also lead to megaloblastic anemia. Thus malabsorption (as in celiac disease), gastrectomy, infiltrative disorders of the bowel (including lymphoma and collagen vascular disease such as scleroderma), infections by the fish tapeworm, and metabolic disorders (such as hyperthyroidism and increased demand for folic acid as in advanced stages of malignancy) all will lead to reduced levels of vitamin B_{12} and folic acid. A deficiency of either vitamin B_{12} or folic acid will lead to maturational arrest of the red cell precursors, which yields large and apparently immature red cell precursors—hence the name *megaloblastic*. The nuclei of red cell precursors are in an immature stage for the maturation of the cytoplasm, which results in an unusually large nucleus. Deficiency in vitamin B_{12} and folic acid leads to abnormalities or inadequate synthesis of DNA, which results in a delayed or blocked mitotic division. There is no abnormality in the synthesis of RNA or cytoplasmic protein, and that portion of the cell continues to mature.

139. The answer is D. *(Wilson, 12/e. pp 463–464.)* The cells shown are eosinophils, and eosinophilic leukocytosis (eosinophilia) is defined as an absolute count exceeding $500/mm^3$. Causes include cutaneous allergic reactions, allergic disorders such as asthma or hay fever, Hodgkin's disease, and parasitic infections (trichinosis, schistosomiasis, strongyloidiasis). Adrenocortical stimulation by administration of corticosteroids may cause eosinophilic leukopenia (eosinopenia), but not eosinophilia. The most common cause of eosinophilia is probably allergy to drugs such as iodides, aspirin, and sulfonamides; eosinophilia is also seen in collagen vascular diseases (rheumatoid arthritis, allergic angiitis). Marked eosinophilia occurs in hypereosinophilic syndromes including Loeffler's syndrome and idiopathic hypereosinophilic syndrome (50,000 to 100,000 eosinophils/mm^3). Corticosteroid therapy induces remission.

140. The answer is D. *(Williams, 4/e. p 1498.)* Hemarthroses do not occur frequently in patients who have von Willebrand's disease and usually are caused by trauma. A prolonged bleeding time affects most of the patients and, together with a moderate deficiency in coagulation factor VIII, is usually acceptable for establishing the diagnosis of von Willebrand's disease. Decreased retention of platelets in glass bead filters, normal numbers of platelets, and menorrhagia are usual findings, but petechiae rarely occur. The most common symptoms include epistaxis and increased susceptibility to bruises.

141. The answer is A. *(Robbins, 4/e. pp 492–494.)* Increased amounts of δ-aminolevulinic acid (ALA) and coproporphyrin are found in the urine of patients who have ingested lead. Lead interferes with erythropoiesis by inhibiting the activity of several enzymes, including δ-ALA synthetase and ALA dehydrase. Thus the various degrees of anemia that are usually associated with lead poisoning are more likely to be mediated by interference with erythropoietic-dependent enzymes than to be the result of hemolysis.

142. The answer is C. *(Robbins, 4/e. pp 739–743.)* The bone marrow aspirate exhibits a proliferation of plasma cells that are characterized by well-defined perinuclear clear zones and by dense cytoplasmic basophilia due to increased RNA accumulations. Weakness, weight loss, recurrent infections, proteinuria, anemia, and abnormal proliferation of plasma cells in the bone marrow are findings that highly suggest the presence of multiple myeloma, a plasma cell dyscrasia. The more definitive diagnostic criteria are findings of M-component in the results of serum electrophoresis and plasma cell levels above 15 percent in the bone marrow. Multiple myeloma, occurring more commonly in males than in females, shows an increasing incidence with increasing age, and most patients are in their seventies.

143. The answer is D. *(Robbins, 4/e. pp 146–149.)* The cell in the photomicrograph is known as Gaucher's cell, the pathognomonic histopathologic finding in Gaucher's disease, and is a histiocyte typically found in the spleen, liver, and bone marrow. The cytoplasm contains glucocerebroside in an increased concentration that is demonstrable by periodic acid–Schiff reagent staining and appears wrinkled or striated in ordinary light microscopy. Histochemical ultrastructure studies have revealed that the unique cytoplasmic wrinkles are due to the presence of many spindle-shaped bodies (Gaucher's bodies) that contain 90 percent glucocerebroside and that show increased acid phosphatase activity. A characteristic histopathologic (but not pathognomonic) finding in Niemann-Pick disease is the foam cell; this cell is found mainly in lymphoid tissues.

144. The answer is B. *(Robbins, 4/e. pp 146–149.)* Gaucher's disease is transmitted through an autosomal *recessive* mechanism. The former view that the disease was transmitted through an autosomal *dominant* mechanism was based on erroneous interpretation of the incidence of the disease in several successive generations. The most commonly occurring of the three types of Gaucher's disease is type I. Patients who have this form can expect to live long lives even though symptoms progressively intensify with advancing age.

145. The answer is C. (*Anderson, 9/e. pp 826–827. Robbins, 4/e. pp 695, 1070.*) A woman who manifests a hemorrhagic diathesis following childbirth should be considered to have intravascular coagulopathy until proof to the contrary is obtained—for instance, the condition may be due to retained products of conception. However, the peripheral blood smear depicted in the question shows, in addition to thrombocytopenia (three to four platelets are normally present in every high-power field), remarkably misshaped red blood cells (poikilocytosis) in the form of schistocytes (fragments of red cells), spherocytes, and, importantly, "helmet" red cells, so named because of their similarity in shape to military or football helmets. Helmet cells imply the presence of microangiopathic hemolytic anemia and are thought to form through hemolytic-mechanical red cell membrane disruption by passing through arteriole-capillary beds that have fibrin thrombin meshes. Disorders that cause microangiopathic hemolytic anemia are childhood and adult hemolytic uremic syndrome and thrombotic thrombocytopenic purpura (TTP). The lack of jaundice and neurologic symptoms in this case rules out TTP. The combination of microangiopathic hemolytic anemia and renal insufficiency strongly suggests hemolytic uremic syndrome.

146. The answer is A. (*Robbins, 4/e. pp 666–670.*) Homozygous expression of hemoglobin S results in nearly all the hemoglobin in the red blood cell's being of the S type. Thus, most of the circulating red cells have the abnormal sickling forms that are sequestered by the spleen and produce sludging within the splenic capillaries and consequent multiple and continuing infarctions. Eventually the spleen becomes small as it is replaced by fibrous tissue. This is sometimes referred to as "autosplenectomy." Multiple crises contribute to this event. Massive enlargements of the spleen may be found in neoplastic blood disorders. Chronic lymphocytic leukemia (CLL) produces some very large spleens late in the disease, but massive splenomegaly has been seen in many examples of leukemias and lymphomas, including hairy cell leukemia. Even conversion from cutaneous T-cell lymphoma (mycosis fungoides) may result in a transformed immunoblastic-like sarcoma state. The syndrome of myelodyspoiesis also results in splenomegaly.

147. The answer is C. (*Robbins, 4/e. pp 708–711.*) The Rappaport classification has separated NHL into nodular and diffuse categories; this is of major importance since the nodular pattern, independent of the cytologic subtype, is associated with a much better prognosis than is the diffuse type. The nodular lymphomas are composed of neoplastic B cells. Unlike the diffuse lymphomas, which often occur in children and adolescents, nodular lymphomas are rare in those under 20. They affect males and females equally, while diffuse lymphomas are much more common in males. Well-differentiated lymphocytic lymphoma and lymphoblastic lymphoma occur only in the diffuse form.

148. The answer is B. *(Williams, 4/e. p 1069.)* First described by Frizzera in 1974 and subsequently described by Lukes and Tindle, immunoblastic lymphadenopathy (IBL), also called *angioimmunoblastic lymphadenopathy with dysproteinemia,* is an interesting systemic illness. It is characterized by hepatosplenomegaly, skin rash, hemolytic anemia, polyclonal hypergammaglobulinemia, "B" symptoms (including fever and weight loss, with some spontaneous remissions, but often terminating in death), and evolution into immunoblastic sarcoma (rare). The lymph nodes show total effacement of their normal architecture by a diffuse proliferation of plasma cells, lymphoid cells, plasmacytoid cells, and immunoblasts. There is a characteristic proliferation of postcapillary venules, with a type of branching called *arborization* (see photomicrograph). PAS-positive lakes of proteinaceous fluid may also be present in the lymph node. The ultimate prognosis is grim.

149. The answer is B. *(Wilson, 12/e. pp 1416–1417.)* The finding of mu heavy-chain proteins in the serum is diagnostic generally of macroglobulinemia and specifically of mu heavy-chain disease. The benign form of macroglobulinemia has been detected in asymptomatic persons without findings of lymphadenopathy, hepatosplenomegaly, anemia, or bone marrow infiltrates of lymphocytes and plasma cells. Increasing levels of the abnormal serum component, onset of bleeding, anemia, or serum hyperviscosity may indicate the need for treatment.

150. The answer is B. *(Robbins, 4/e. p 717.)* T-cell lymphomas occurring in the thoracic cavity in young patients usually arise in the mediastinum and have a particularly aggressive clinical course with rapid growth in the mediastinum impinging upon the trachea or mainstem bronchi and leading to marked respiratory deficiency, which can in turn lead to death in a relatively short period of time if not treated. These unique lymphomas are characterized by rapid cell growth and spread into the circulation, where they produce elevated total white counts reflected by circulating lymphoma cells. As T cells they have characteristics of rosette formation with sheep blood cells. T cells also have subtypes and subsets, which can be delineated by monoclonal antibodies as CD4 helper, CD8 suppressor (cellular differentiation) T-cell surface antigens. The tumor cells also express IL-2 receptor. FC receptors occur on B cells and macrophages. Class II HLA antigens can be found on macrophages, Langerhans cells, and dendritic reticulum cells.

151. The answer is E. *(Henry, 18/e. pp 630, 641–642.)* Seen in the photomicrograph are sideroblasts that are demonstrating distinctive rings of Prussian blue–positive granules that indicate iron. Approximately 35 percent of normoblasts in normal bone marrow contain ferritin granules under normal conditions of iron metabolism. Heme synthetase mediates the attachments of iron onto protoporphyrin for the synthesis of hemoglobin. In sideroblastic anemia the production of globin or of heme is markedly reduced because of the deficiency of pyridoxine and ferritin, which contains iron accumulations with sideroblasts without progression into hemoglobin. The accumulation of these ferritin granules takes place in the mitochondria, where heme synthetase is located, and then can be seen rimming the nucleus of the normoblast—hence the name *ring sideroblasts*. This is the opposite abnormality from iron deficiency anemia. This type of anemia may be seen in patients suffering from alcoholism, selective deficiencies of pyridoxine, and in malignant conditions such as breast carcinoma.

152. The answer is D. *(Robbins, 4/e. pp 686–688.)* Intravascular iron is bound to transferrin, which is usually about 33 percent saturated with iron. Increased saturation occurs in states of iron overload (hemochromatosis), in severe liver disease, hemolytic conditions, and marrow hypoplasia (reduced iron utilization). Iron deficiency is associated with low serum iron levels, increased iron-binding capacity, and decreased saturation.

153. The answer is D. *(Henry, 18/e. pp 657, 670.)* Both thalassemia minor and iron deficiency anemia are microcytic disorders in which the mean corpuscular hemoglobin is usually found to be reduced. Red blood cell indexes may be useful in differentiating the two disorders, for while the mean corpuscular hemoglobin concentration (MCHC) is often normal or only slightly reduced in association with thalassemia minor, the MCHC is often definitely reduced in association with iron deficiency anemia. Both pernicious and folate deficiency anemias lead to megaloblastic changes in erythrocytes.

154. The answer is D. *(Robbins, 4/e. pp 737–739.)* Myeloid metaplasia with myelofibrosis is a myeloproliferative disorder in which the bone marrow is hypocellular and fibrotic and extramedullary hematopoiesis occurs, mainly in the spleen (myeloid metaplasia). Marked splenomegaly with trilinear proliferation of normoblasts, immature myeloid cells, and large megakaryocytes occurs. Giant platelets and poikilocytic (teardrop) red cells are seen in the peripheral smear. Clinically, myeloid metaplasia may be preceded by polycythemia vera or chronic myeloid leukemia. Biopsy of the marrow is essential for diagnosis. In contradistinction to chronic myeloid leukemia, levels of leukocyte alkaline phosphatase are elevated or normal in myeloid metaplasia; in CML, levels are low or absent. In 5 to 10 percent of cases of myeloid metaplasia, acute leukemia occurs. In aplastic anemia the marrow is very hypocellular, but consists largely of fat cells, not fibrosis. There is no splenomegaly. Microangiopathic and other hemolytic anemias that result from trauma to red cells show many erythrocytic abnormalities (helmet and burr cells, triangle cells, and schistocytes) in the peripheral smear.

155. The answer is C. (*Robbins, 4/e. pp 261, 288–289, 728–729.*) Chronic myeloid leukemia (CML) is one of the four chronic myeloproliferative disorders, but, unlike myeloid metaplasia or polycythemia vera, CML is associated with the Philadelphia chromosome translocation t (9;22) in over 90 percent of cases. Association with the translocation t (8;14) is characteristic of Burkitt's lymphoma. In differentiating CML from a leukemoid reaction, several other features are important: lack of alkaline phosphatase in granulocytes, increased basophils in the peripheral blood, and, often, increased platelets in early stages followed by thrombocytopenia in late or blast stages. Other well-known features of CML include marked splenomegaly, leukocyte counts greater than 50,000/mm^3, and mild anemia.

156. The answer is C. (*Anderson, 9/e. pp 494–495.*) While the exact interactions between different cells are not totally understood, there is current evidence that an initiating antigen is first processed by a macrophage. The macrophage interacts with helper T cells and B cells in a conceptual triangular fashion with helper T cells functioning in the recognition of the carrier component of the antigen on the macrophage as well as recognizing the major histocompatibility complex (MHC) marker (Ia) on the macrophage surface. The macrophage appears to concentrate the antigen, thereby orchestrating interactions between itself and the T and B lymphocytes. After stimulation, the B cell may differentiate into antibody-producing plasma cells. Eosinophils and basophils function in type I reactions (anaphylaxis) by degranulation and binding of IgE.

157. The answer is C. (*Robbins, 4/e. pp 714–715, 718.*) The large-cell immunoblastic lymphoma is one of the three high-grade lymphomas, which also include lymphoblastic lymphoma and small, noncleaved lymphomas, such as Burkitt's lymphoma. Lymphoblastic lymphoma occurs predominantly in adolescents, is closely related to T-cell acute lymphoblastic leukemia, and, in addition to a mediastinal mass, disseminates early to bone marrow and blood. In contrast, large-cell immunoblastic lymphoma is predominantly of B-cell origin (5 to 10 percent are T cell) and occurs in much older people, many of whom had a prior immune or lymphoproliferative disorder (Sjögren's syndrome, AIDS, or renal transplant immunosuppression). Bone marrow involvement is uncommon except in late stages; extranodal tumor (retroperitoneum) is common. The tumor is aggressive and rapidly fatal if untreated. The cells appear plasmacytoid (B immunoblasts) or show multilobed, polymorphous nuclei (T immunoblasts), but molecular studies are essential to differentiate T-cell receptor gene rearrangement from the immunoglobulin gene rearrangements of B immunoblasts.

158. The answer is B. (*Robbins, 4/e. pp 223, 267.*) The findings given are consistent with Wiskott-Aldrich syndrome. The Pelger-Huët anomaly involves leukocytes that have dumbbell-shaped nuclei but function normally. Some of the listed clinical features occur in the Chédiak-Higashi syndrome, but delayed hypersensitivity reactions are normal. In chronic granulomatous disease, leukocytes are unable to kill phagocytized bacteria, but delayed hypersensitivity reactions and platelet counts are normal. In patients who have Hodgkin's disease, a different constellation of symptoms occurs.

159. The answer is D. (*Robbins, 4/e. pp 677–678.*) The autoimmune hemolytic anemias are important causes of acute anemia in a wide variety of clinical states and can be separated into two main types: those secondary to "warm" antibodies and those reactive at cold temperatures. Warm-antibody autoimmune hemolytic anemias react at 37°C in vitro, are composed of IgG, and do not fix complement. They are found in patients with malignant tumors, especially leukemia-lymphoma; with use of such drugs as alpha methyldopa; and in the autoimmune diseases, especially lupus erythematosus. Cold-antibody autoimmune hemolytic anemia reacts at 4 to 6°C, fixes complement, is of the IgM type, and is classically associated with mycoplasma pneumonitis (pleuropneumonia-like organisms). These antibodies are termed *cold agglutinins* and may reach extremely high titers and cause intravascular red cell agglutination.

160. The answer is C. (*Robbins, 4/e. pp 717–722.*) The diagnosis of Hodgkin's disease depends on the total histologic picture and the presence of binucleated or bilobed giant cells with prominent acidophilic "owl-eye" nucleoli known as Reed-Sternberg cells. However, cells similar in appearance to Reed-Sternberg cells may also be seen in infectious mononucleosis, mycosis fungoides, and other conditions. Thus, while Reed-Sternberg cells are necessary for histologic confirmation of the diagnosis of Hodgkin's disease, they must be present in the appropriate histologic setting of lymphocyte predominance, nodular sclerosis, mixed cellularity, or lymphocyte depletion.

161. The answer is E. *(Robbins, 4/e. pp 323–325.)* Infectious mononucleosis is a benign lymphoproliferative disorder caused by the Epstein-Barr virus (EBV). It typically occurs in young adults and presents with systemic symptoms, lymphadenopathy, and pharyngitis. Hepatosplenomegaly may be present. Peripheral blood shows an absolute lymphocytosis, and many lymphocytes are atypical with irregular nuclei and abundant basophilic vacuolated cytoplasm. These represent CD8-positive T-killer cells induced by EBV-transformed B lymphocytes. These atypical lymphocytes are usually adequate for diagnosis. The heterophil test (increased sheep red cell agglutinin) is usually positive, but virus-specific EBV antibodies are more specific. Administration of ampicillin for a mistaken diagnosis of streptococcal pharyngitis results in a rash in many patients.

162. The answer is E. *(Robbins, 4/e. pp 735–736. Williams, 4/e. pp 193–200.)* Polycythemia rubra vera (PRV) is one of the myeloproliferative diseases characterized by excessive proliferation of erythroid, granulocytic, and megakaryocytic precursors derived from a single stem cell. In PRV the erythroid series dominates, but there is hyperplasia of all elements. There is plethoric congestion of all organs. The liver and spleen are typically moderately enlarged and may show extramedullary hemopoiesis. Thrombotic complications are an important cause of morbidity and mortality, and major and minor hemorrhagic complications are also frequent. The red cell count is elevated with hematocrit >60 percent. The white cell count and platelet count are also elevated. Leukocyte alkaline phosphatase (LAP) activity is elevated in contrast to chronic myeloid leukemia, where it is reduced.

163–167. The answers are: 163-C, 164-C, 165-D, 166-A, 167-B. *(Robbins, 4/e. pp 724–730.)* Auer rods are often prominent in the hypergranular promyelocytes of acute promyelocytic leukemia since they are formed from the abnormal azurophilic granules. Myeloblasts predominate in acute myeloblastic leukemia (AML) and, therefore, only a few granules, or occasional Auer rods, are present. Acute promyelocytic leukemia is associated with a short course and widespread petechiae and ecchymoses, cutaneous or mucosal, from disseminated intravascular coagulation. The M1 and M3 classes refer to the French-American-British (FAB) classification of AML: M1 is AML in which myeloblasts predominate and M3 is acute promyelocytic leukemia with promyelocytes numerous. Myeloperoxidase is present in both, especially in M3.

AML occasionally follows chemotherapy and radiotherapy for Hodgkin's disease.

Chronic lymphocytic leukemia occurs most frequently after the age of 50 (90 percent of cases). It is associated with long survival in many cases and the few symptoms are related to anemia and the absolute lymphocytosis of small mature cells. Splenomegaly may be noted. Some patients are asymptomatic.

Acute lymphoblastic leukemia (ALL) affects children and young adults with marked lymphadenopathy, some splenomegaly, and hepatomegaly. Since chemotherapy at present results in complete remission in 90 percent of children, with more than 50 percent alive 5 years later, it is essential to differentiate ALL from acute myeloblastic leukemia in which prognosis is poor. Cytochemical differentiation includes PAS-positive blasts in most cases of ALL and the presence of terminal deoxynucleotidyl transferase (TdT) in 95 percent of cases of ALL, but in less than 5 percent of acute myeloblastic leukemias.

Hairy cell leukemia and chronic lymphocytic leukemia (CLL) are considered to be chronic lymphoproliferative disorders. CLL is a neoplasm of B cells, like most other lymphoid malignancies. Through molecular analysis, hairy cells are now known to rearrange and express immunoglobulin genes, assigning them also to B-cell lineage.

168–170. The answers are: 168-E, 169-C, 170-A. (*Robbins, 4/e. pp 287–289. Williams, 4/e. pp 89–92, 202–205, 1068.*) Chromosomal translocations are present in some malignancies, which suggests they have a possible role in malignant transformation. In some cases the translocation has been shown to involve proto-oncogenes, which raises the possibility of proto-oncogene activation. Eighty to ninety percent of cases of follicular non-Hodgkins lymphoma contain the t14;18 translocation. In these cases the immunoglobulin heavy chain locus is the site of a translocation involving the *bcl*-2 proto-oncogene on chromosome 18 with consequent overexpression of the *bcl*-2 protein.

More than 90 percent of cases of chronic myeloid leukemia exhibit the Philadelphia chromosome, a reciprocal translocation from the long arm of chromosome 22 to chromosome 9. The segment of chromosome 9 involved in translocation contains the proto-oncogene c-*abl*, which is rearranged in proximity to a break point cluster region *(bcr)* on chromosome 22. The resultant chimeric c-*abl/bcr* gene encodes a protein with tyrosine kinase activity.

More than 90 percent of cases of Burkitt's lymphoma have a translocation involving the c-*myc* proto-oncogene on chromosome 8 and the immunoglobulin heavy chain locus on chromosome 14. This change results in activation of the c-*myc* oncogene and overexpression of its gene product.

171–174. The answers are: 171-C, 172-A, 173-D, 174-B. *(Robbins, 4/e. pp 210–220.)* Amyloid is a pathologic proteinaceous substance deposited in various body sites in a variety of disease processes. Many chemically distinct classes of amyloid fibril exist, each derived from a chemically related precursor protein. Amyloid light chain (AL) is the most common amyloid protein and is derived from immunoglobulin light chains. It is deposited in various immunocyte dyscrasias, most commonly multiple myeloma and including nodular malignant lymphoma.

Amyloid-associated (AA) protein is a polypeptide derived from serum amyloid-associated protein, which is produced in the liver. Systemic deposits of AA protein occur in reactive systemic amyloidosis, which complicates various chronic infectious and inflammatory processes, most commonly rheumatoid arthritis and including other connective tissue diseases, bronchiectasis, and inflammatory bowel disease.

Beta$_2$ amyloid protein is a polypeptide that forms the amyloid found in the cores of cerebral plaques and in the blood vessels in Alzheimer's disease.

Transthyretin is a normal serum protein that binds and transports thyroxine and retinol. A mutant form of this protein is deposited as amyloid in both familial amyloid polyneuropathies and senile cardiac amyloidosis.

Cardiovascular System

175. An 82-year-old woman complaining of headaches, visual disturbances, and muscle pain has a biopsy of the temporal artery. The changes revealed by the biopsy specimen are shown in the photomicrograph below. The next course of action is to

(A) administer corticosteroids
(B) verify with a repeat biopsy
(C) administer anticoagulants
(D) perform angiography
(E) order an erythrocyte sedimentation rate (ESR) test

176. If the coronary arteries on dissection at autopsy show severe atherosclerosis in a patient who had clinical acute (60-h) myocardial infarction, you would expect to find

(A) definite gross evidence of infarction
(B) coronary thrombosis in 90 percent of cases
(C) coronary thrombosis in 65 percent of cases
(D) a plaque with ulceration, fissure, or hemorrhage
(E) rupture of a papillary muscle

177. Complete obliteration of the aortic lumen by a coarctation proximal to the ductus arteriosus is fatal unless

(A) the foramen ovale is closed
(B) the ductus is ligated
(C) pulmonary stenosis coexists
(D) the ductus remains patent
(E) the tricuspid valve is incompetent

178. Which of the following conditions is most likely to predispose to thrombosis and embolism?

(A) Atrial fibrillation
(B) Pulmonary stenosis
(C) Ventricular septal defect
(D) Aortic stenosis
(E) Atrial septal defect

179. Features of Fallot's tetralogy include all the following EXCEPT

(A) obstruction to the pulmonary outflow
(B) hypertrophy of the right ventricle
(C) aortic dextroposition in 50 percent of cases
(D) cyanosis developing before 1 year of age
(E) ventricular septal defect

180. The form of vascular disease responsible for malignant hypertension is

(A) medial calcific sclerosis
(B) arteriosclerosis obliterans
(C) hyperplastic arteriolosclerosis
(D) hyaline arteriolosclerosis
(E) thromboangiitis obliterans

181. The most common cause of infectious myocarditis is

(A) diphtheritic infection
(B) Coxsackie viral infection
(C) Chagas' disease
(D) trichinosis
(E) brucellosis

182. The mortality from myocardial infarction is most closely related to the occurrence of

(A) a pericardial effusion
(B) pulmonary edema
(C) coronary artery thrombosis
(D) an arrhythmia
(E) systemic hypotension

183. A synonym for *nonbacterial thrombotic endocarditis* is

(A) atypical verrucous endocarditis
(B) marantic endocarditis
(C) Libman-Sacks endocarditis
(D) viridans endocarditis
(E) none of the above

184. The pathology evident in the photomicrograph below usually first appears after which of the following lengths of time following a myocardial infarction?

(A) 12 h
(B) 3 days
(C) 7 days
(D) 14 days
(E) 28 days

185. An elderly man treated for congestive heart failure for years with digitalis and furosemide dies of pulmonary edema. A postmortem examination of the heart would most likely show

(A) severe left ventricular hypertrophy
(B) right and left ventricular hypertrophy
(C) right ventricular infarction
(D) aortic and mitral valve stenosis
(E) a dilated, globular heart with thin walls

186. The photomicrograph below depicts the presence of

(A) disseminated candidiasis
(B) pigmented purpuric dermatosis
(C) anaphylactoid purpura (leukocytoclastic angiitis)
(D) erythema multiforme
(E) reaction to the bite of an arthropod

187. Manifestations of rheumatic fever that are of major diagnostic value include all the following EXCEPT

(A) subcutaneous nodules
(B) migratory arthritis of large joints
(C) fever
(D) erythema marginatum
(E) chorea minor

188. Bacterial endocarditis constitutes the greatest threat to patients who have which of the following forms of congenital heart disease?

(A) Atrial septal defect
(B) Ventricular septal defect
(C) Pulmonic stenosis
(D) Tetralogy of Fallot
(E) Patent ductus arteriosus

189. A 56-year-old woman died in a hospital where she was being evaluated for shortness of breath, ankle edema, and mild hepatomegaly. Because of the gross appearance of the liver at necropsy in the photograph below, one would also expect to find

(A) a pulmonary saddle embolus
(B) right heart dilatation
(C) portal vein thrombosis
(D) biliary cirrhosis
(E) splenic amyloidosis

190. The necrotizing inflammation of the small gastrointestinal artery shown in the photomicrograph below is most likely due to

(A) myasthenia gravis
(B) polyarteritis nodosa
(C) atherosclerosis
(D) dissecting aneurysm
(E) syphilis

191. Unexpected sudden cardiac death is a very rare complication of

(A) severe coronary artery disease
(B) myocarditis
(C) cardiac tamponade
(D) mitral valve prolapse
(E) dilated or hypertrophic cardio-myopathy

192. Major risk factors associated with development of coronary and generalized atherosclerosis (AS) include all the following EXCEPT

(A) cigarette smoking
(B) elevated high-density lipoprotein (HDL) levels
(C) diabetes mellitus
(D) hypertension
(E) hypercholesterolemia

193. The biopsy specimen shown below reveals a dermal vascular tumor with angular, slitlike spaces and spindle cells in the dermal stroma. This lesion is associated with all the following EXCEPT

(A) four clinically distinct forms
(B) intestinal bleeding
(C) depletion of T-suppressor cells
(D) early histologic resemblance to dermatitis
(E) tumor origin from vascular endothelium

194. Following development of an acute myocardial infarction (MI), the LEAST likely complication is

(A) cardiac arrhythmia
(B) cardiogenic shock
(C) ventricular aneurysm
(D) cardiac rupture
(E) thromboembolism

195. Acute infective endocarditis differs from subacute endocarditis in all the following respects EXCEPT

(A) the time required for the lesion to develop
(B) the nature of the preponderant organism
(C) embolization and dissemination
(D) the nature of valvular vegetations
(E) the causative organism

196. Severe mitral stenosis, as shown in the photograph below, is frequently accompanied by all the following EXCEPT

(A) aortic valve disease
(B) antecedent rheumatic fever
(C) left atrial enlargement with atrial fibrillation
(D) pulmonary valvular stenosis
(E) chronic passive pulmonary congestion

197. Cardiac involvement has been linked to all the following conditions EXCEPT

(A) hemochromatosis
(B) Rocky Mountain spotted fever
(C) sarcoidosis
(D) breast carcinoma
(E) early gastric cancer

198. The most frequent cause of aortic valve incompetence and regurgitation is

(A) latent syphilis
(B) infective endocarditis
(C) rheumatic fever
(D) aortic dissection
(E) congenital

199. The heart in the gross photograph below came from a patient who

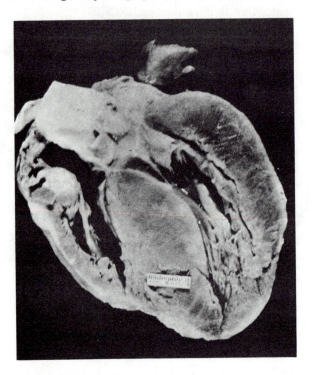

(A) suffered from alcohol toxicity
(B) had Libman-Sacks endocarditis
(C) may have had a family history of similar cardiac involvement
(D) frequently had obstructive symptoms
(E) had a hypocontractile heart

---

200. Tumors known for involvement of the atrium include all the following EXCEPT

(A) angiosarcoma
(B) primary myxoma
(C) lung carcinoma
(D) prostatic carcinoma
(E) renal cell carcinoma

DIRECTIONS: Each group of questions below consists of lettered headings followed by a set of numbered items. For each numbered item select the one lettered heading with which it is **most** closely associated. Each lettered heading may be used **once, more than once, or not at all.**

Questions 201–204

Match the following descriptive phrases with the appropriate lettered type of cardiomyopathy.

(A) Hypertrophic cardiomyopathy
(B) Dilated (congestive) cardiomyopathy
(C) Constrictive (restrictive) cardiomyopathy
(D) Secondary cardiomyopathy
(E) Endomyocardial fibrosis

201. Thirty percent of patients are prone to sudden cardiac death

202. May develop in patients with multiple myeloma

203. Obstruction of left ventricular outflow of blood

204. Usually identified in Southeast Asia and Africa

Questions 205–208

For each cardiac condition choose the infectious agent with which it is most likely to be associated.

(A) Coxsackievirus
(B) *Mycobacterium tuberculosis*
(C) *Streptococcus*
(D) *Treponema*
(E) *Escherichia coli*

205. Primary myocarditis

206. Rheumatic fever

207. Aortic aneurysms

208. Suppurative pericarditis

Questions 209–212

For each aneurysm, choose the disease or syndrome with which it is most likely to be associated.

(A) Ehlers-Danlos syndrome
(B) Kawasaki's disease
(C) Rheumatic disease
(D) Polycystic renal disease
(E) Takayasu's arteritis

209. Berry aneurysm

210. Dissecting aortic aneurysm

211. Coronary aneurysm

212. Abdominal and distal thoracic aortic aneurysms

Questions 213–217

Match each disorder below with the most appropriate cardiovascular abnormality.

(A) Libman-Sacks disease
(B) Coarctation of the aorta
(C) Fiedler's myocarditis
(D) Patent ductus arteriosus
(E) Thromboembolism
(F) Fibrosis of tricuspid and pulmonary valves

213. Prosthetic heart valves

214. Congenital rubella

215. Turner's syndrome

216. Systemic lupus erythematosus

217. Carcinoid syndrome

Cardiovascular System
Answers

175. The answer is A. (*Robbins, 4/e. pp 574–576.*) Giant-cell arteritis (temporal arteritis), although not a major public-health problem, is an important disease to consider in the differential diagnosis of patients of middle to advanced age who present with a constellation of symptoms that may include migratory muscular and back pains (polymyalgia rheumatica), dizziness, visual disturbances, headaches, weight loss, anorexia, and tenderness over one or both of the temporal arteries. The cause of the arteritis (which may include giant cells, neutrophils, and chronic inflammatory cells) is unknown, but the dramatic response to corticosteroids suggests an immunogenic origin. The disease may involve any artery within the body, but involvement of the ophthalmic artery or arteries may lead to blindness unless steroid therapy is begun. Therefore, if clinically suspected, the workup to document temporal arteritis should be expedited and should include a biopsy of the temporal artery. Frequently, the erythrocyte sedimentation rate (ESR) is markedly elevated to values of 90 or greater. Whereas tenderness, nodularity, or skin reddening over the course of one of the scalp arteries, particularly the temporal, may show the ideal portion for a biopsy, it is important to recognize that temporal arterial segments may be segmentally uninvolved or not involved at all even when the disease is present.

176. The answer is D. (*Robbins, 4/e. pp 564, 606–608.*) At autopsy, coronary artery thrombosis has been found in less than 50 percent of cases of myocardial infarction (MI). However, when coronary angiography is done within 4 h of MI onset, a thrombosed artery is found in almost 90 percent of cases; occlusion is found in only about 60 percent when angiography is delayed for 12 to 24 h. Therefore, lysis occurs or there is relaxation of spasm, or both. Also, intravenous or intracoronary fibrinolysins restore flow to thrombosed arteries in more than 75 percent of recent MIs. These findings are proof of coronary thrombosis, whether it is found at autopsy or not. Ulcerated, fissured, or hemorrhagic atheromas are usually found beneath the thrombus, whether still attached or lysed.

177. The answer is D. (*Robbins, 4/e. pp 624–625.*) Coarctation of the aorta occurs in 6 to 14 percent of cases of congenital heart disease. In its infantile form, coarctation takes place in the root of the aorta proximal to the ductus arteriosus, which, if patent, serves as a bypass to allow blood flow to the arterial system. Usually, surgical intervention is necessary for infants who have this anomaly, which may cause death soon after birth or within the first year of life.

178. The answer is A. *(Robbins, 4/e. pp 99–106.)* Stasis of blood in fibrillating atria predisposes to thrombosis and embolism. Systemic embolization from left atrial thrombi may cause infarction in the brain, lower extremities, spleen, and kidneys. Endocardial mural thrombi occur as a consequence of myocardial infarction, bacterial endocarditis, or nonbacterial (marantic) endocarditis.

179. The answer is C. *(Wilson, 12/e. p 932.)* Fallot's tetralogy consists of subaortic ventricular septal defect, obstruction to right ventricular outflow, aortic override of the ventricular septal defect, and moderate right ventricular hypertrophy. The obstruction to right ventricular outflow may be caused by infundibular stenosis of the right ventricle or stenosis of the pulmonic valve. A right-sided aorta occurs in about 25 percent of cases with tetralogy. Most patients are cyanotic from birth or develop cyanosis by the end of the first year of life, since even mild obstruction to right ventricular outflow is progressive. Tetralogy of Fallot is the most common cause of cyanosis after 1 year of age and causes 10 percent of all forms of congenital heart disease. Hypoxic attacks and syncope are serious complications, forming the commonest mode of death from this disease during infancy and childhood. Other complications include infectious endocarditis, paradoxical embolism, polycythemia, and cerebral infarction or abscess.

180. The answer is C. *(Robbins, 4/e. pp 569–570, 577.)* *Malignant hypertension* refers to dramatic elevations in systolic and diastolic blood pressure often resulting in early death from cerebral and brainstem hemorrhages. Pathologically the renal vessels demonstrate a concentric obliteration of arterioles by an increase in smooth muscle cells, and protein deposition in a laminar configuration that includes fibrin material, which leads to total and subtotal occlusion of the vessels. Hyaline arteriolosclerosis as seen in diabetes is presumably caused by leakage of plasma components across the endothelium with or without hypertension. Medial calcific sclerosis (Mönckeberg's arteriosclerosis) is characterized by dystrophic calcification in the tunica media of muscular arteries. Thromboangiitis obliterans (Buerger's disease) is occlusion by a proliferative inflammatory process in arteries of heavy cigarette smokers and is often associated with HLA-A9, B5 genotypes.

181. The answer is B. *(Anderson, 9/e. pp 659–664. Robbins, 4/e. pp 640–643.)* Although numerous agents—bacterial, protozoal, fungal, or parasitic—cause infectious myocarditis, the most common type is viral myocarditis, which often presents as a primary infection. The Coxsackie viral group, principally Coxsackie B, is most often implicated. Coxsackie myocarditis in children is often preceded by upper respiratory tract infection. Other viral diseases in which myocarditis occurs include rubella and polio. Chagas' disease *(Trypanosoma cruzi)* is also prominent as a cause of myocarditis in endemic areas of South America, where up to half the population is infected. Bacterial myocarditis is not common, but the diphtheria bacillus is causative through its exotoxin (toxic myocarditis). The bacteria of brucellosis, tularemia, and tuberculosis produce small granulomas within the myocardium. *Trichinella spiralis* larvae frequently penetrate myocardial fibers; they do not encyst, but interstitial myocarditis may result.

182. The answer is D. *(Robbins, 4/e. pp 612–614.)* In myocardial infarction, life-threatening arrhythmias occur in approximately 45 percent of patients without shock and in more than 90 percent of patients with shock. The most common arrhythmias are expressed as ventricular extrasystoles, but atrial extrasystoles, sinus tachycardia, and sinus bradycardia also occur. Even without arrhythmias, nearly two-thirds of patients with acute myocardial infarcts develop heart failure and pulmonary edema. Sudden death (death within 24 h of onset of symptoms and signs) occurs in about 20 to 25 percent of acute attacks.

183. The answer is B. *(Anderson, 9/e. pp 652–655.)* Nonbacterial thrombotic endocarditis is a form of endocarditis involving the mitral and aortic valves especially, characterized by resemblance to the verrucous-like protuberances of rheumatic valvulitis, which are usually large and friable; smooth and polypoid and shaggy forms are also encountered. These also may resemble the vegetations of bacterial endocarditis, but the lesions are sterile and contain no microorganisms. Both surfaces of the valves are not involved, as they may be in Libman-Sacks or atypical verrucous endocarditis. *Viridans endocarditis* is a synonym for *subacute bacterial endocarditis.* Nonbacterial thrombotic endocarditis is also referred to as *terminal* or *marantic endocarditis* and is associated in this country with advanced stages of cachexia, such as found in advanced malignancy or starvation. It occurs in many other terminal wasting diseases but has recently been described in well-nourished persons who have died acutely; thus, the older terms *marantic* and *terminal* are probably not appropriate. The pathogenesis is not clear, although there is evidence for increased coagulability in some patients, and the disorder may be associated with disseminated intravascular coagulation.

184. The answer is B. *(Robbins, 4/e. pp 609–611.)* Usually by 3 days after a myocardial infarction, the predominant microscopic features that develop and that can be seen in a stained section of the affected myocardium include co-agulation necrosis of fibers and evidence of extensive neutrophilic exudation. Interstitial edema may also be observed in microscopy, and the cross-striations of fibers may appear less recognizable. In gross examination 3 days after the infarction, the infarct has a hyperemic border surrounding a central portion that is yellow-brown and soft as the result of fatty change.

185. The answer is E. *(Robbins, 4/e. pp 598–601.)* The morphologic changes of clinical congestive heart failure cannot always be correlated with necropsy findings of the heart because there may be hypertrophy, dilatation, a combination of both, or even an absence of both. Many patients with long-standing congestive heart failure after decompensation will have hearts that are maximally dilated, with thinned and unusually soft myocardium rather than hypertrophic ventricular myocardium. This thinning of the myocardium occurs after a long period of compensatory hypertrophy and reflects a state in which the capacity of the myocardium to compensate has been exceeded. The first response of the myocardium to a demand for increased work (load) is to undergo hypertrophy according to Starling's law, leading to an increase in stroke volume. Eventually, this mechanism is exceeded under states of increased oxygen demand or demand for more cardiac output, and cardiac decompensation results, with the worst complication being acute pulmonary edema as a consequence of left ventricular failure.

186. The answer is C. *(Robbins, 4/e. pp 573–574.)* Anaphylactoid purpura (also known as leukocytoclastic or hypersensitivity angiitis) is characterized clinically by palpable purpura in patients reacting to an antigen derived from drugs (especially the semisynthetic penicillins), from infections (including beta-streptococcal pharyngitis), and possibly from neoplasms. Pathologically, the epidermis is generally intact with vascular damage in the form of fibrinoid necrosis and occlusion of these small capillaries, venules, and arterioles of the dermis by fibrin and proteinaceous deposits, which may include IgA and complement. Hallmarks of the disease histologically are neutrophils that extend out from the damaged vessels and show karyorrhexis (nuclear dust). Extravasated red cells are also seen. Disseminated candidiasis is characterized by varying degrees of severity of epidermal micropustules, folliculitis, or dermal abscesses. Erythema multiforme generally presents with epidermal cell necrosis, an inflammatory cell infiltrate in the dermis, and bullae separating the epidermis from the dermis. Arthropod reactions may have polymorphic inflammatory cells that include neutrophils, eosinophils, macrophages, and lymphocytes, but lymphocytic hyperplasia is frequently the hallmark in the hypersensitivity chronic form.

187. The answer is C. *(Robbins, 4/e. pp 629–633.)* Rheumatic fever (RF) is a systemic disease with the major findings of migratory polyarthritis of large joints, carditis, erythema marginatum of skin (although skin involvement is not very common), subcutaneous nodules, and Sydenham's chorea, a neurologic disorder with involuntary, purposeless, rapid movements, most likely to occur in adolescent females and during pregnancy. There is no relation to Huntington's chorea. Fever is a minor characterization, although quite frequent. Rheumatic nodules may develop over pressure points during the later stages and seldom occur in cases without cardiac involvement. RF usually follows a pharyngeal infection with group A β-hemolytic streptococci because of an autoimmune mechanism based on cross-reactions between cardiac antigens and antibodies evoked by one of the many streptococcal antigens, e.g., streptococcal M protein. Immunofluorescence shows immunoglobulins and complement along sarcolemmal sheaths of cardiac myofibers, but Aschoff bodies seldom contain immunoglobulins or complement.

188. The answer is B. *(Robbins, 4/e. pp 633–637.)* Even though children and infants who have small isolated ventricular septal defects are usually asymptomatic, and even though two-thirds of infants who have uncomplicated lesions will have spontaneous closure of their ventricular septal defects by the age of 5, the main risk for these patients is bacterial endocarditis. Protection against bacteremia with antibiotics during routine but potentially infectious procedures is therefore required.

189. The answer is B. *(Robbins, 4/e. pp 600–601.)* The photograph shows the classic pattern of hepatic congestion around central veins, which leads to necrosis and degeneration of the hepatocytes surrounded by pale peripheral residual parenchyma. This is the pattern arising in the liver from chronic passive congestion as a result of right heart failure ("nutmeg liver"). Mitral stenosis with consequent pulmonary hypertension leads to right heart failure, as does any cause of pulmonary hypertension, such as emphysema (cor pulmonale). Right heart failure also leads to congestion of the spleen and transudation of fluid into the abdomen (ascites) and lower extremity soft tissues (pitting ankle edema) as a result of venous congestion. Portal vein thrombosis is most often seen in association with hepatic cirrhosis.

190. The answer is B. *(Robbins, 4/e. pp 571–573.)* Polyarteritis nodosa, as a necrotizing inflammation that occurs in episodes at random locations within or on the walls of medium-sized and small arteries, has been reported in about

0.1 percent of autopsies and affects, in order of increasing frequency, the arteries associated with peripheral and central nerves, skeletal muscles, pancreas, gastrointestinal tract, liver, heart, and kidneys. Proceeding in stages, the inflammatory reaction features acute necrosis, with fibrinoid deposition and neutrophilic infiltration, and leads to thrombosis of the lumen and destruction of the internal elastic membrane. Polyarteritis nodosa probably could be more accurately called "panarteritis nodosa," because *all* vascular coats are subject to inflammation. A remnant of the internal elastic membrane is visible in the photomicrograph.

191. The answer is D. *(Wilson, 12/e. p 945.)* The most common cause of sudden death in the adult is cardiac arrhythmia (usually ventricular fibrillation) due to severe coronary artery disease, with or without acute myocardial infarction. Ventricular fibrillation is also often due to primary cardiomyopathy, myocarditis, or congestive heart failure. However, sudden death is a rare complication of mitral valve prolapse (MVP), floppy valve syndrome, or the systolic click-murmur syndrome. In MVP the major complication is mitral insufficiency with left ventricular failure; however, MVP is asymptomatic in the majority of patients. Echocardiography has shown MVP to be common (5 to 10 percent of the general population). It is usually of unknown cause, but 10 to 15 percent of cases are familial with autosomal dominant inheritance. It is fairly frequent in Marfan's syndrome or cystic medial necrosis. There is excess mitral valve tissue and elongated chordae and the echocardiogram shows posterior displacement of the posterior (rarely anterior) mitral leaflet late in systole. Another interesting, but rare, noncardiac cause of sudden unexpected death is unrecognized anaphylaxis from insect stings. Postmortem sera should be examined for elevated venom-specific IgE antibodies, and laryngeal and pulmonary edema noted at autopsy.

192. The answer is B. *(Anderson, 9/e. pp 618–621. Robbins, 4/e. pp 557–562.)* Hypercholesterolemia (serum cholesterol greater than 200 to 230 mg/dL) is one of the major risk factors for development of atherosclerosis. Hypercholesterolemia is associated with elevated low-density lipoprotein (LDL), which contains a high proportion of cholesterol. Men with cholesterol levels above 240 mg/dL have a threefold risk of death from myocardial infarct, compared with men with cholesterol below 200. However, in contrast to the LDL fraction, the HDL fraction is inversely related to the incidence of coronary heart disease (CHD). The Framingham heart study found that low plasma levels of HDL are a potent risk factor for coronary artery disease. HDL levels are increased by exercise, small amounts of alcohol, and administration of estrogens, but cigarette smoking depresses plasma HDL levels.

193. The answer is C. *(Robbins, 4/e. pp 591–592, 1291–1292.)* Kaposi's sarcoma (KS) comprises four distinct forms. The classic, or European, form has been known since 1862. It occurs in older men of Eastern European or Mediterranean origin (predominantly Italian or Jewish) and is characterized by purple maculopapular skin lesions of the lower extremities and visceral involvement in only 10 percent of cases. The African form occurs in younger people and is more aggressive; it often involves lymph nodes in children. The rare form in immunosuppressed recipients of renal transplants often regresses when immunosuppression stops. In the epidemic form associated with AIDS, skin lesions may occur anywhere and include dissemination to mucous membranes, GI tract, lymph nodes, and viscera. Histologic determination is difficult, but all four clinical types appear similar. Early, irregular, dilated epidermal vascular spaces, extravasated red cells, and hemosiderin (like granulation tissue or stasis dermatitis) are characteristic. Later, more characteristic lesions show spindle cells around slit-spaces that are angular and contain red cells—a picture like that of angiosarcoma. The tumor cells are almost certainly of vascular endothelial origin (blood vessel or lymphatic or both). This often multifocal disease is rarely fatal, but death may be caused by frequent opportunistic infections or, less often, lymphoma, leukemia, or myeloma. There is depletion of T-helper cells, but T-suppressor cells are normal or increased.

194. The answer is D. *(Robbins, 4/e. pp 609, 613.)* Cardiac rupture, whether of free wall, septum, or papillary muscle, occurs in only 1 to 5 percent of cases following acute myocardial infarction. It occurs usually within the first week of infarction when there is maximal necrosis and softening (4 to 5 days) and is very rare after the second week. Rupture of the free wall results in pericardial hemorrhage and cardiac tamponade. Rupture of the interventricular septum causes a left-to-right shunt. Serious mitral valve incompetence results from rupture of anterior or posterior papillary muscles. Other common complications include arrhythmias such as heart block, sinus arrhythmias, or ventricular tachycardia or fibrillation. These occur in 90 percent of complicated cases. Next in importance, but not in frequency (only 10 percent), is cardiogenic shock from severe left ventricular contractile incompetence. Milder left ventricular failure with lung edema occurs in 60 percent, while mural thrombosis with peripheral emboli may occur in up to 40 percent. Ventricular aneurysm forms a "bulge" of the left ventricular chamber; it consists of scar tissue, does not rupture, but may contain thrombus.

195. The answer is D. *(Robbins, 4/e. pp 633–637.)* Infective endocarditis, unlike rheumatic endocarditis, continues to be a clinical problem even in the antibiotic era, with such new factors as intravenous drug abuse and immunosuppression contributing to its persistence. The successful outcome of treatment is directly dependent on early recognition and diagnosis, since with time the infective organisms (such as yeast, bacteria, rickettsiae) tend to be covered with fibrin and platelets, thereby preventing access of antibiotics to the organisms. In addition, delayed treatment allows time for local valvular destruction. Acute endocarditis (AC) tends to develop within days on previously normal valves (60 percent of cases), whereas subacute endocarditis (SEC) takes more time to develop, may be clinically silent, and may be manifested only by the patient's complaint of not being "up to par." The organism causing AC tends to be pathogenic (e.g., *Staphylococcus aureus* or gonococcus); the organism causing SEC tends to be relatively innocuous (e.g., microaerophilic streptococci, *Streptococcus viridans,* and even diphtheroids). Bacterial embolization from the valves to other organs occurs mainly in AC and is much less common in SEC. Despite small differences, such as the smaller vegetations occurring in SEC than in AC, it is not usually possible to distinguish SEC vegetations from AC vegetations through only structural criteria.

196. The answer is D. *(Anderson, 9/e. pp 672–673.)* Mitral stenosis is most often associated with aortic valve disease and occasionally with tricuspid valve disease, especially in people with antecedent rheumatic fever. Occasionally, both aortic and mitral disease result from atherosclerosis. Pulmonary valvular stenosis is rarely caused by either aortic or mitral disease. Since severe mitral stenosis prevents significant regurgitation, left ventricular enlargement would not be expected. Left atrial enlargement and chronic pulmonary congestion are common in mitral disease.

197. The answer is E. *(Anderson, 9/e. pp 660–661, 686, 704–705.)* The heart is frequently involved in hemochromatosis with brownish discoloration of the myocardium; diffuse, severe involvement results in a soft, brown, dilated organ with marked dilatation of the right ventricle and vena cava. Hemosiderin granules in myocardial fibers and myocardial fibrosis are evident. Heart failure or arrhythmias due to hemosiderin in conduction system fibers may occur. Rickettsial diseases are frequently complicated by myocarditis, especially in scrub typhus and in about 50 percent of cases of epidemic typhus and Rocky Mountain spotted fever. Rickettsiae cause a systemic vasculitis that forms the basis for the interstitial myocarditis and other lesions. Sarcoidosis is now recognized as a cause of heart disease, even without the existence of cor pulmonale. Formation of sarcoid granulomas may be accompanied by considerable fibrosis, myocardial damage, heart failure, and sudden death. More often, cor pulmonale results from extensive lung involvement. Metastatic malignancy is the most common tumor to involve the heart, especially the pericardium, by vascular dissemination or direct extension. The primary tumor is most frequently carcinoma of lung or breast, lymphoma, leukemia, or malignant melanoma. Tumor involvement of pericardium frequently causes hemorrhagic effusion. In early gastric cancer, tumor has invaded no further than the submucosa.

198. The answer is C. *(Anderson, 9/e. pp 650–652, 675–676.)* Aortic regurgitation (AR) is rheumatic in origin in approximately 70 percent of cases. Much less frequently it is due to syphilis, ankylosing spondylitis (rarely), infective endocarditis, aortic dissection, or aortic dilatation from cystic medial necrosis. Congenital forms of aortic stenosis occur fairly frequently but AR is rarely congenital in origin. In chronic AR, patients remain asymptomatic for many years, but clinical manifestations will include exertional dyspnea, angina, and left ventricular failure. Owing to the rapidly falling arterial pressure during late systole and diastole, there is often wide pulse pressure, Corrigan's "water-hammer" pulse, capillary pulsations at the nail beds, and a pistol-shot sound over the femoral arteries. A blowing diastolic murmur is heard along the left sternal border. Volume overload of the heart is the basic defect and results in left ventricular dilatation and hypertrophy.

199. The answer is C. *(Robbins, 4/e. pp 644–646.)* The cardiomyopathy shown in the photograph is designated *hypertrophic cardiomyopathy* with the synonyms of *idiopathic hypertrophic subaortic stenosis (IHSS), hypertrophic obstructive cardiomyopathy,* and *asymmetric septal hypertrophy (ASH).* It is characterized by a prominent and hypertrophic interventricular septum that is out of proportion to the thickness of the left ventricle. Histologically the myocardial fibers have disarray caused by wide fibers with unusual orientation, and prominent hyperchromatic nuclei. There is increased incidence within families and there is evidence that it may be an autosomal dominant disorder. Patients may have dyspnea, light-headedness, and chest pain, especially upon physical exertion; however, many patients appear to be asymptomatic although a sudden, unexpected death occurs not infrequently, especially following or during physical exertion. There may be abnormalities of the coronary arteries. The mitral valve may be thickened and patients may experience endocarditis on it. Cardiac output can be markedly reduced in some patients because of reduced volume of the left ventricle. As the patient ages, however, cardiac dilatation often improves the reduced left ventricular volume. Chronic alcoholism and a flabby, hypocontractile heart occur with dilated (congestive) cardiomyopathy.

200. The answer is D. *(Robbins, 4/e. pp 651–653.)* The benign myxoma most often arises in the left atrium and is the most common primary cardiac tumor. It may involve any cardiac chamber but is three to four times more common in the left atrium, may be small or large, is attached to the endocardium, and often produces a ball-valve action with prolapse through the mitral valve during diastole. Systemic emboli are frequent to brain, heart, and kidneys and consist of fragments of myxoma. Most myxomas are sporadic, but some are familial with autosomal dominant inheritance and associated pigmented nevi, nodular adrenal hyperplasia, breast fibroadenoma, and testicular and pituitary tumors. Renal cell carcinoma may involve the renal vein and extend into the inferior vena cava and into the right atrium. Rarely, cardiac symptoms caused by this venous extension may be the first sign of renal tumor. Sarcoma (most frequently angiosarcoma) is the most common primary malignant cardiac tumor and usually originates in the right atrium or pericardium. Metastatic tumors of the heart are much more frequent than primary tumors, and bronchogenic and breast carcinomas are the most common sources. Prostatic carcinoma produces osteoblastic bone metastases.

201–204. The answers are: 201-A, 202-C, 203-A, 204-E. *(Robbins, 4/e. pp 643–648.)* The cardiomyopathies (CMP) may be classified into primary and secondary forms. The primary forms are mainly idiopathic (unknown cause). The causes of secondary CMP are many and range from alcoholism (probably the most common cause in the United States) to metabolic disorders to toxins and poisons. Whereas there are not many gross organ and microscopic anatomic features of CMP, a few rather characteristic hallmarks are well recognized in separating the types. However, extensive clinical, historical, and laboratory data contribute as much if not more to classification of the type of CMP present than does biopsy or even the postmortem heart examination.

Hypertrophic CMP encompasses those cases in which the major gross abnormality is to be found within the interventricular septum, which is usually thicker than the left ventricle. If there is obstruction of the ventricular outflow tract, there will be moderate hypertrophy in the left ventricles as well, but the septum usually remains thicker, yielding an appearance of asymmetric hypertrophy. This form of CMP occurs in families (rarely sporadically) and is thought to be autosomal dominant. Up to one-third of these patients have been known to die sudden cardiac deaths, often under conditions of physical exertion. Histologically, the myofibers interconnect at angles and are hypertrophied.

In dilated (congestive) CMP, the ventricular chambers are markedly dilated, with the walls either of normal thickness or thinner than normal. Whereas many idiopathic cases exist, some patients have a history of heavy alcohol intake. The microscopic appearance is not distinctive. The ventricles may have mural thrombi.

Constrictive (restrictive) CMP is associated in the United States with amyloidosis and endocardial fibroelastosis and is so named because the infiltration and deposition of amyloid in the endomyocardium and the layering of collagen and elastin over the endocardium affect the ability of the ventricles to accommodate blood volume during asystole. The heart is more likely to be so involved if the systemic amyloidosis is associated with primary systemic or plasma cell tumors (myeloma). Endocardial fibroelastosis occurs mainly in infants and in the first 1 to 2 years of life and causes a prominent fibroelastic covering to form over the endocardium of the left ventricle. There may be associated aortic coarctation, ventricular septal defects, mitral valve defects, and other abnormalities.

Endomyocardial fibrosis is a form of restrictive CMP found mainly in young adults and children in Southeast Asia and Africa, where it accounts for a not insignificant number of deaths in these age groups. It differs from endocardial fibroelastosis in the United States in that elastic fibers are not present. Its cause is totally unknown.

205–208. The answers are: 205-A, 206-C, 207-D, 208-B. *(Anderson, 9/e. pp 650–652, 659–661, 778–780.)* Primary myocarditis, an isolated lesion that is not secondary to a generalized disease, is most commonly caused by such agents as type B coxsackievirus, echoviruses, and *Toxoplasma gondii.*

Streptococci are generally considered the causative agents of rheumatic fever; and although group A β-hemolytic streptococci are most strongly implicated, viruses continue to be suspected as among the causes of this systemic nonsuppurative inflammatory disease. Abundant evidence supports the view that antibodies generated in the immunologic reaction to infection with group A β-hemolytic streptococcus cross-react with myocardial fibers, smooth muscle cells, and connective tissue glycoproteins. Aschoff bodies, produced in response to this cross-reaction, are regarded as pathognomonic for rheumatic fever.

Aortic aneurysms of luetic carditis constitute the tertiary manifestation of syphilis and become evident 15 to 20 years after persons have contracted infection with *Treponema pallidum.* Elastic tissue and smooth muscle cells of the media undergo ischemic destruction as a result of the treponemal infection. As a consequence of ischemia in the media, musculoelastic support is lost, leading to aortic aneurysms, widening of the aortic valve ring, and narrowing of the coronary ostia.

Suppurative pericarditis is a form of acute pericarditis that can be caused by *Mycobacterium tuberculosis* and is considered to invariably denote entry into the pericardium of bacterial, mycotic, or parasitic agents. In the suppurative pericarditis caused by *M. tuberculosis* (tuberculous pericarditis), tuberculosis of the mediastinal nodes has been a finding in the majority of affected adults. Up to 500 mL of thick fluid (typical of caseation necrosis) containing granulocytes, erythrocytes, and, in 50 percent of patients who have tuberculous pericarditis, tubercle bacilli may be found in the pericardium.

209–212. The answers are: 209-D, 210-A, 211-B, 212-E. *(Anderson, 9/e. pp 774–775. Robbins, 4/e. pp 155–157, 576–579, 1020–1021.)* Berry aneurysms in the circle of Willis have been noted in about one-sixth of patients with adult polycystic renal disease. Subarachnoid hemorrhage from these, because of hypertension, accounts for death in about 10 percent of patients with adult polycystic renal disease.

Ehlers-Danlos syndromes (EDSs) are a group of eight syndromes characterized by defects in collagen synthesis. In EDS IV there is deficient synthesis of type III collagen and a tendency to rupture of muscular arteries, including dissecting aneurysms of the aorta. A high incidence of dissecting aneurysm also occurs in Marfan's syndrome and it may occur in coarctation of the aorta.

Both Takayasu's and Kawasaki's diseases (mucocutaneous lymph node syndrome) are examples of arteritis. Kawasaki's disease is thought to be an immune complex disorder, possibly caused by *Propionibacterium acnes,* although a retrovirus has been suggested. It was first recognized in Japan, but there have been several outbreaks in the continental U.S. and in Hawaii. A skin rash, lymphadenopathy, arthritis, and arteritis are predominant. Coronary arteritis results in aneurysms and is associated with myocarditis and sometimes infarction. The disease characteristically affects boys under 4 years old.

Takayasu's arteritis, or "pulseless disease," is most common in young women and affects large and medium arteries, especially the aorta and its larger branches. Aneurysms are common in the abdominal and distal thoracic aorta, especially in older patients. There may be thrombosis of vessels arising from the aortic arch and many cases demonstrate the aortic arch syndrome. Marked weakening of the pulses in the upper extremities is noted. This arteritis has been known as *aortic arch syndrome, primary aortitis,* and *giant-cell arteritis of the aorta,* in addition to other synonyms. Arteriosclerotic aneurysms are also common in the abdominal aorta; syphilitic aneurysm is practically limited to the thoracic segment.

213–217. The answers are: 213-E, 214-D, 215-B, 216-A, 217-F. *(Anderson, 9/e. pp 652–653, 731–735, 741–743.)* Congenital rubella contracted in the first trimester of pregnancy may result in any of several malformations, including patent ductus arteriosus (PDA), pulmonic stenosis, ventricular septal defect, and cataracts, as well as deafness. PDA accounts for about 10 to 15 percent of all congenital heart disease, while ventricular septal defect is the most common form with an incidence of 20 to 30 percent. In pregnancy, a rising IgM antibody titer indicates recent or primary infection by rubella virus. Secondary infection occurs rarely, after vaccination, but there is only a rise in the IgG (not IgM) antibody level, and fetal infection does not occur.

Turner's syndrome, characterized by short stature and hypogonadism (chromosomal abnormality 45,XO), is fairly common; 10 to 20 percent of patients with this syndrome have coarctation of the aorta. Coarctation accounts for about 10 to 15 percent of all congenital heart disease.

Nonbacterial verrucous endocarditis (Libman-Sacks disease) involves valvular lesions associated with systemic lupus erythematosus (SLE). They consist of very small, warty deposits on any valve, especially the mitral and aortic, and are located on the surface exposed to the forward flow of the blood. Pancarditis, especially pericarditis or pericardial effusion, is more common in SLE.

Prosthetic heart valves predispose to cerebral embolism and patients with artificial/mechanical valves have more risk of embolism than those with tissue valves. Unfortunately, degeneration and subsequent valve dysfunction are more common with bioprostheses, and about 25 percent of these require replacement within 10 years.

Fibrosis of tricuspid and pulmonary valve cusps, resulting in tricuspid insufficiency and pulmonic stenosis, occurs in some patients with the carcinoid syndrome, probably because of 5-hydroxytryptamine from the carcinoid tumor.

Respiratory System

DIRECTIONS: Each question below contains five suggested responses. Select the **one best** response to each question.

218. Horner's syndrome is associated with

(A) lymphangitis carcinomatosa
(B) bronchial carcinoid
(C) exophthalmos
(D) tumor of the superior sulcus
(E) thoracocervical venous dilatation

219. Alpha$_1$-antitrypsin deficiency is associated with

(A) thalassemia
(B) nephrotic syndrome
(C) panlobular emphysema
(D) centrilobular emphysema
(E) anthracosis

220. Human infection caused by the dog heartworm, *Dirofilaria immitis,* may cause

(A) bronchitis
(B) subcutaneous nodules
(C) thoracic lymphadenopathy
(D) conjunctival infection
(E) pulmonary infarction

221. A young woman succumbed after an 8-month course of severe dyspnea, fatigue, and cyanosis that followed an uneventful delivery of a healthy infant. At necropsy, small atheromas were present in the large and small branches of the pulmonary arteries. Which of the following findings can be predicted in the histologic slides of the lungs?

(A) Diffuse hemorrhage and infarctions
(B) Diffuse alveolar hyaline membranes
(C) Severe atelectasis and edema
(D) Marked medial hypertrophy of pulmonary arterioles
(E) Multiple pulmonary emboli

222. Which of the following bronchogenic carcinomas is associated with production of parathormone-like substances?

(A) Acinar adenocarcinoma
(B) Papillary adenocarcinoma
(C) Bronchioloalveolar carcinoma
(D) Squamous cell carcinoma
(E) Oat cell carcinoma

223. The cells in the photomicrograph below appeared in a cytologic specimen of sputum from a 52-year-old man with chest pain, some loss of weight, and a nonproductive cough of 8 months' duration. Which of the following is the most likely diagnosis?

(A) Oat cell (small cell undifferentiated) carcinoma
(B) Adenocarcinoma
(C) Squamous cell carcinoma
(D) Squamous metaplasia
(E) *Pneumocystis* pneumonia

224. A patient hospitalized for fractures of the long bones who develops mental dysfunction, increasing respiratory insufficiency, and renal failure should be suspected of having

(A) fat embolism syndrome
(B) disseminated intravascular coagulopathy
(C) myocardial infarction
(D) aortic valve disease
(E) respiratory distress syndrome

225. The major pathologic injury in interstitial lung disease is generally accepted to be

(A) diffuse pneumonia
(B) bronchopneumonia
(C) bronchiolitis
(D) bronchitis
(E) alveolitis

226. A 48-year-old woman with a 26-pack-year history of cigarette smoking was noted to have abnormal cells (malignancy is suspected) in sputum cytology. The chest x-ray is presented (right). What is the most likely diagnosis?

(A) Sarcoidosis
(B) Adenocarcinoma
(C) Breast carcinoma
(D) Small cell carcinoma
(E) Squamous cell carcinoma

227. The organism that is most likely to cause the necrotizing pulmonary lesion shown in the photomicrograph below is

(A) *Pseudomonas aeruginosa*
(B) *Mycobacterium tuberculosis*
(C) *Pneumocystis carinii*
(D) *Trichinella spiralis*
(E) *Candida albicans*

228. Acute lymphoblastic leukemia was diagnosed in a 10-year-old child. When this child later developed a patchy pulmonary infiltrate and respiratory insufficiency, a lung biopsy was performed. The material obtained by biopsy was then stained with Gomori's methenamine-silver stain and is shown in the photomicrograph below. In consideration of the patient's signs and microscopic evaluations, the prognosis is now complicated by

(A) *Pseudomonas* pneumonia
(B) *Aspergillus* pneumonia
(C) *Pneumocystis carinii* pneumonia
(D) pneumococcal pneumonia
(E) influenza pneumonia

229. Common tumors or cysts in the superior mediastinum include

(A) schwannoma
(B) bronchogenic cyst
(C) thymoma
(D) neurofibroma
(E) pericardial cyst

230. A 45-year-old man presents with shortness of breath, cough with mucoid sputum, and some weight loss and has diffuse, bilateral alveolar infiltrates on chest roentgenogram. Pulmonary function tests reveal decreased diffusing capacity and hypoxemia. The patient had worked for several years at grinding aluminum. The photomicrograph below is from a lung biopsy. Your diagnosis is

(A) *Pneumocystis carinii* pneumonia
(B) diffuse alveolar damage (DAD)
(C) pulmonary edema
(D) pulmonary alveolar proteinosis (PAP)
(E) lipid pneumonia

231. True statements about the molecular biology of lung tumors include all the following EXCEPT

(A) K-*ras* oncogenes are activated in many adenocarcinomas
(B) epidermoid cancers express high levels of receptor for transforming growth factor
(C) the receptor expressed by epidermoid cancers is produced by the c-*erbB* oncogene
(D) small cell carcinomas show a deletion in the short arm of chromosome 3
(E) abnormal retinoblastoma antioncogenes are common in adenocarcinoma

232.   The condition seen below in the gross photograph of a sagittal section
of the lung may occur in which of the following?

(A) Squamous cell carcinoma
(B) Oat cell carcinoma
(C) Malignant mesothelioma
(D) Benign spindle cell mesothelioma
(E) Metastatic carcinoma

233.   The most common benign tumor of the lung is the

(A) fibroma
(B) hemangioma
(C) hamartoma
(D) leiomyoma
(E) carcinoid

234. The photomicrograph of the bronchial washing specimen shown below depicts

(A) Schaumann bodies
(B) ferruginous bodies
(C) cholesterol crystals
(D) *Candida* species
(E) silica particles

---

235. Which is the most useful single immunohistochemical marker in differentiating pulmonary adenocarcinoma from mesothelioma?

(A) Leu-M1
(B) Antivimentin
(C) S-100
(D) Carcinoembryonic antigen (CEA)
(E) Cytokeratin

Questions 236–237

Shown in the photomicrograph below is a section of alveolar tissue that was taken at autopsy of a 4-day-old premature infant.

236. The pathologic process that is evident is consistent with

(A) pneumococcal pneumonia
(B) congenital pulmonary cystic malformation
(C) extralobar pulmonary sequestration
(D) primary fungal pneumonitis
(E) respiratory distress syndrome (hyaline membrane disease)

237. A similar histopathologic condition can be seen in lungs of adults who have all the following conditions EXCEPT

(A) viral pneumonia
(B) uremia
(C) pulmonary irradiation
(D) severe bacterial infection
(E) tuberculosis

DIRECTIONS: Each group of questions below consists of lettered headings followed by a set of numbered items. For each numbered item select the **one** lettered heading with which it is **most** closely associated. Each lettered heading may be used **once, more than once, or not at all.**

Questions 238–241

Match the most characteristic finding with each respiratory disorder.

(A) Myasthenic syndrome
(B) Fungal infection
(C) Hemorrhagic interstitial pneumonitis
(D) Nasal mucosal ulcerations
(E) Asthmatic bronchitis

238. Wegener's granulomatosis

239. Oat cell carcinoma

240. Byssinosis

241. Goodpasture's syndrome

Questions 242–244

For each tumor, choose its most common site of origin.

(A) Nasal cavity
(B) Neuroendocrine cells of bronchi
(C) Submucosal bronchial glands
(D) Terminal bronchioles
(E) Bronchial blood vessels

242. Bronchial carcinoid

243. Bronchioloalveolar carcinoma

244. Adenoid cystic carcinoma

Questions 245–248

Match the pathologic or clinical findings with the appropriate organism.

(A) *Coccidioides immitis*
(B) Pathogenic staphylococci
(C) Type 3 pneumococci
(D) *Nocardia asteroides*
(E) *Legionella pneumophila*

245. Diarrhea and delirium with pneumonia

246. Acid-fast and aerobic presentation

247. Hypersensitivity reactions

248. Exotoxin production

Respiratory System
Answers

218. The answer is D. *(Robbins, 4/e. pp 801–804.)* Horner's syndrome occurs with apical (superior sulcus) tumors of any type (Pancoast tumor). The syndrome is characterized by enophthalmos, ptosis, miosis, and anhidrosis on the same side as the lesion due to invasion of the cervical sympathetic. Involvement of the brachial plexus causes pain and paralysis in the ulnar nerve distribution. Venous dilatation of the upper thorax and neck is seen in the superior vena caval syndrome because of compression or invasion by lung cancer or lymphoma. Lymphangitic carcinomatosis usually results from spread of metastatic tumors within subpleural lymphatics.

219. The answer is C. *(Robbins, 4/e. pp 137, 159, 767–770.)* Patients who are homozygous for alpha$_1$-antitrypsin deficiency develop severe panlobular emphysema, often before the age of 40. This genetic disorder accounts for about 10 percent of cases of emphysema. Other factors in the pathogenesis of emphysema include air pollution and smoking. The disorder results from any variant of the numerous alleles on the chromosomal loss of Pi (proteinase inhibitor). Cigarette smoking greatly accelerates the emphysema in the homozygous (Pi ZZ) state.

220. The answer is E. *(Robbins, 4/e. pp 419–420.)* Pulmonary dirofilariasis is caused by a single larva of the dog heartworm, *D. immitis,* which embolizes from the right heart to a peripheral pulmonary artery and causes a small infarct. This nodular, or "coin," lesion may be mistaken for a tumor. Histologically, granulomatous or mixed inflammation borders infarcted lung with a central dead, or degenerate, larva. The lesion should be excluded when a necrotic lung nodule is found at surgery, but multiple sections may be needed to find the larva. Animal filariae such as *D. immitis* or *D. tenuis* (which usually infects raccoons) are arthropod-borne. *D. tenuis* may cause conjunctival and skin infections including subcutaneous nodules. North American *Brugia* (which generally infects raccoons and lynx) involves lymphatics and causes enlargement of one cervical/thoracic lymph node.

221. The answer is D. *(Robbins, 4/e. pp 764–765.)* Many pathologic pulmonary changes can be found in the lungs of patients who expire under conditions of progressive, unexplained dyspnea, fatigue, and cyanosis. These changes range from pulmonary fibrosis to hypersensitivity pneumonitis and to recurrent, multiple pulmonary emboli. Furthermore, traditional hospital treatment modalities for progressive pulmonary deterioration (including high oxygen delivery, overhydration, lack of pulmonary ventilation, irregular ventilation by mechanical respiratory assistance [PEEP], and superimposed nosocomially acquired pneumonitis) can complicate pulmonary pathologic findings. However, unremitting, progressive dyspnea, cyanosis, and fatigue in a young woman should suggest the diagnosis of primary pulmonary hypertension. Pulmonary vascular sclerosis is always associated with pulmonary hypertension primary or secondary to other states, such as emphysema and mitral stenosis.

222. The answer is D. (*Robbins, 4/e. pp 294–296, 801.*) Squamous cell carcinoma, the most frequent type of bronchogenic carcinoma (25 to 30 percent), is the type most often associated with hypercalcemia. The hypercalcemia may be related to osteolytic bone metastases, but hypercalcemia as a paraneoplastic syndrome may occur in the absence of skeletal metastases. This form of hypercalcemia is caused by tumor production of parathormone-like substances, or prostaglandin E, or other calcium-mobilizing tumor products such as growth factors involved in the histogenesis of the tumor. These probably bind to the parathyroid hormone receptors in bone to mimic the calcium-mobilizing action of parathormone. Hypercalcemia is rare with oat cell tumors, which are much more likely to produce ACTH-like (Cushing's syndrome) or ADH-like substances.

223. The answer is C. (*Takahashi, 2/e. pp 305–306.*) The cells shown have rather bizarre shape, marked nuclear hyperchromasia and irregularity, an increase in nuclear area and in nucleocytoplasmic ratio, and marked variation in cell size and shape—all criteria suggestive of malignancy. Malignant cells of this type (often with orangeophilic cytoplasm) found in sputum are diagnostic of squamous cell carcinoma. In adenocarcinoma the cells form clusters and have less hyperchromatic nuclei but prominent nucleoli and vacuolated cytoplasm. Oat cell carcinoma has much smaller cells and tight clusters with nuclear molding. *Pneumocystis* is seen as a very fine, bubbly or frothy (pink) organism in sputum.

224. The answer is A. (*Robbins, 4/e. pp 110–111.*) Fat embolism syndrome can supervene as a complication within 3 days following severe trauma to the long bones. However, the pathogenesis must be regarded as unknown because simple entrance of microglobular fat into the circulation as a result of damage to small vessels in marrow tissue occurs in over 90 percent of patients with trauma and bone fracture, yet the syndrome occurs in only a minority of such patients. Laboratory and clinical findings can simulate those of intravascular coagulopathy, which may be a component of fat embolism syndrome, with a major difference of split products of fibrin seen mainly in intravascular coagulopathy. Plasma levels of free fatty acids are elevated in fat embolism and may contribute to pulmonary vascular alterations. At autopsy fat material can be demonstrated in fat stains of frozen sections of lung, brain, and kidney in patients who had the syndrome.

225. The answer is E. *(Robbins, 4/e. pp 789–791.)* In diffuse interstitial lung disease (ILD) the early and major event is damage to the alveolar walls. First, an interstitial inflammation affects mainly the septae (interstitial alveolitis) with edema of the alveolar walls and an infiltrate of lymphocytes and monocyte-macrophages. The alveolar lining cells (mostly type I) are injured or become necrotic and are replaced by proliferating type II cells creating a cuboidal epithelial lining; alveolar endothelial cells are also injured, allowing exudation of fluid into the interstitium. If reversal does not occur, the changes become chronic with eventual fibrous scarring of alveolar walls, impaired respiratory function, and pulmonary hypertension. Causes of ILD include occupational exposure to inorganic dust (asbestos, silica), gases, aerosols, and organic dust, in addition to drugs (bleomycin, busulfan, nitrofurantoin) and infections (cytomegalovirus and tuberculosis). The major interstitial lung diseases of unknown cause include sarcoidosis and idiopathic pulmonary fibrosis (Hamman-Rich syndrome).

226. The answer is D. *(Anderson, 9/e. pp 1011–1013.)* The chest x-ray in this clinical example demonstrates a central mass in the region of the hilum of the right lung. The differential diagnosis of a radiographic central mass includes consideration of undifferentiated small cell carcinoma, sarcoidosis, lymphoma, and, less commonly, other forms of bronchogenic carcinoma. In sputum cytology, small cell carcinomas demonstrate clusters of lymphocyte-like tumor cells in strands, with adjacent tumor nuclei indentation (nuclear molding). The incidence of carcinoma of the lung in males is dropping somewhat, but the overall incidence continues because of greater numbers of women taking up the cigarette habit in recent years, with many of these women starting in their teens. As a consequence, small cell (oat cell) carcinoma is being seen with greater frequency in women.

227. The answer is E. *(Anderson, 9/e. pp 411–413.)* Gomori's methenamine-silver staining technique emphasizes the pseudohyphae and yeast forms of *Candida* species. The pattern of vessel invasion is characteristic of many pathogenic fungi, including *Candida*. Such infections tend to occur in immunologically suppressed patients with other severe, usually neoplastic, diseases.

228. The answer is C. *(Anderson, 9/e. p 948.)* Infection by the protozoan *Pneumocystis carinii* is characterized by the presence of oval and helmet-shaped organisms whose capsules are made more visible by use of Gomori's methenamine-silver staining technique. This organism, although it has low virulence, is opportunistic, for it is often seen to attack severely ill, immunologically depressed patients.

229. The answer is C. *(Robbins, 4/e. pp 803–804.)* The superior mediastinum consists of structures cephalad to the pericardial reflection of the heart. Metastatic carcinoma is fairly frequent in the superior mediastinum, arising often from lung or breast primaries, and less frequently from testis or kidney. Bronchogenic and pericardial cysts occur in the middle mediastinum, whereas neurogenic tumors such as neurofibroma and schwannoma are in the posterior mediastinum. Thymoma is found in the anterosuperior mediastinum. Lymphoma, especially Hodgkin's disease, is common in all mediastinal compartments and involves paratracheal lymph nodes in the superior mediastinum. Seminoma and metastatic choriocarcinoma from the testis are not uncommon. Parathyroid tumors and thyroid lesions occupy both the superior and anterior mediastinum. Retrosternal extension of a goiter, presenting as a superior mediastinal mass, is not unusual.

230. The answer is D. *(Robbins, 4/e. pp 401–402, 759–762, 795–796.)* The alveolar spaces contain an intensely eosinophilic, proteinaceous, granular substance. Alveolar walls are relatively normal without inflammatory exudate or fibrosis, although type II pneumocytes may be hyperplastic. The process is often patchy, with groups of normal alveoli alternating with groups of affected alveoli. Acicular (cholesterol) clefts and densely eosinophilic bodies (necrotic cells) are found within the granular material. Distinction from edema fluid may be difficult, but PAP alveolar material stains with periodic acid–Schiff (PAS). At low power, alveolar material seen in *P. carinii* pneumonia may also mimic PAP, but with high power the foamy material seen with *Pneumocystis* is not present in PAP. In PAP the material is surfactant accumulation, either because of overproduction or failure of macrophage clearance. Causes of PAP include occupational exposure to silica or aluminum dusts. It also occurs in immunosuppressed patients and toxic drug reactions and is often associated with infections like nocardia, fungi, and TB (possible impaired macrophage killing). The treatment of choice is bronchoalveolar lavage to remove the proteinaceous debris.

231. The answer is E. *(Anderson, 9/e. pp 603, 1015.)* Epidermoid carcinomas express high levels of receptor for transforming growth factor (alpha and epidermal GF). This receptor has tyrosine kinase activity and may be permanently attuned to growth or may fail to respond to normal controls. It is produced by the c-*erbB* oncogene. Abnormalities of retinoblastoma antioncogenes are common in small cell carcinoma and atypical carcinoid. Several chromosomal deletions are common in small cell cancer, but the short-arm deletion in chromosome 3 is paramount, while amplification of c-*myc* oncogene is associated with very aggressive behavior. Activation of the K-*ras* oncogene may play a role in pathogenesis of adenocarcinoma of the lung.

232. The answer is C. *(Robbins, 4/e. pp 800, 806–808.)* Malignant mesothelioma and adenocarcinoma are two neoplasms that may involve the pleural surfaces as seen in the gross photograph. Malignant mesothelioma arises from the pleural surfaces and is thus a pleural neoplasm developing in association with significant and chronic exposure to asbestos, usually occupationally incurred. As the malignant mesothelioma spreads, it lines the pleural surfaces including the fissures through the lobes of the lungs and results in a tight and constricting encasement. This restricts the excursions of the lungs during ventilation. Adenocarcinoma of the lung also may invade the pleural surfaces and spread in an advancing manner throughout the pleural lining surfaces. The differential diagnosis histologically between an epithelial type of malignant mesothelioma and an adenocarcinoma may be dufficult and sometimes impossible without special techniques. Oat cell carcinoma usually arises in the central portions of the lungs near the hilum and does not invade the pleura in a spreading fashion. Benign spindle (fibrous) mesothelioma of the lung arises as a discrete mass that is spherical to ovoid in shape in a subpleural configuration and expands as this localized mass without spread over the surfaces.

233. The answer is C. *(Anderson, 9/e. pp 573, 1015–1017, 1020–1021.)* Pulmonary hamartomas, although infrequent, are still the most common of all benign lung tumors. Hamartomas consist of various tissues normally found in the organ where they develop, but in abnormal amounts and arrangement. In the lung, they consist of lobules of connective tissue often containing mature cartilage, fat, or fibrous tissue and separated by clefts lined by entrapped respiratory epithelium. The peak incidence is at age 60, and the tumor is usually found as a well-circumscribed, peripheral, "coin" lesion on routine chest x-ray. Unless the radiographic findings are pathognomonic of hamartoma with "popcorn ball" calcifications, the lesion should be excised or at least carefully followed. Conservative excision is curative.

Bronchial carcinoids are tumors of low-grade malignancy with neuroendocrine differentiation confirmed by immunostaining for neuron-specific enolase, serotonin, calcitonin, or bombesin. They form intrabronchial polypoid growths but most of the tumor mass lies outside the bronchus. Most arise in central bronchi but 20 percent arise in small bronchi and appear as peripheral lung nodules. Surgical excision is curative in at least 90 percent, but 10 percent of carcinoids are aggressive with local invasion or metastases.

234. The answer is B. *(Anderson, 9/e. pp 235, 587, 1003.)* The segmented or beaded, often dumbbell-shaped bodies are ferruginous bodies that are probably asbestos fibers coated with iron and protein. The term *ferruginous body* is applied to other inhaled fibers that become iron-coated; however, in a patient with interstitial lung fibrosis or pleural plaques, ferruginous bodies are probably asbestos bodies. The type of asbestos mainly used in America is chrysotile, mined in Canada, and it is much less likely to cause mesothelioma or lung cancer than is crocidolite (blue asbestos), which has limited use and is mined in South Africa. Cigarette smoking potentiates the relatively mild carcinogenic effect of asbestos. Laminated spherical (Schaumann) bodies are found in granulomas of sarcoid and chronic berylliosis.

235. The answer is D. *(Ordóñez, Am J Surg Pathol 13:276–291, 1989. Robbins, 4/e. pp 807–808.)* The differentiation of pleural mesothelioma from lung adenocarcinoma may be difficult, particularly with the papillary or epithelial type of mesothelioma. Electron microscopy (EM) may not be definitive, although the presence of long, slender microvilli and numerous tonofilaments in mesothelioma contrasts with the short, plump microvilli of adenocarcinoma. Immunocytochemical analysis with the combined use of several antibodies gives more accurate differential diagnosis. More than 90 percent of adenocarcinomas react with carcinoembryonic antigen (CEA) and only adenocarcinomas stain for monoclonal antibody Leu-M1 or S-100 protein. CEA is the most useful single marker to distinguish adenocarcinoma from mesothelioma, which shows complete lack of staining for CEA and Leu-M1. Thus, combined use of several antibodies—especially to CEA and Leu-M1—plus EM, chest radiographs, and adequate biopsy is most valuable in differential diagnosis of lung adenocarcinoma and mesothelioma.

236. The answer is E. *(Anderson, 9/e. pp 838–839.)* The photomicrograph shows classic hyaline membranes coating alveolar sacs and ducts and is diagnostic of the respiratory distress syndrome of the newborn. The eosinophilic, fibrinlike material is related to the alveolar surfactants. Atelectasis is usually also present, especially in premature infants. The deposited material appears not to form in utero, as it is found in infants who have breathed and is not found in stillborns. There is a direct correlation, however, between severity and the degree of prematurity.

237. The answer is E. *(Anderson, 9/e. pp 925–926.)* The presence of hyaline membranes indicates a diagnosis of acute alveolar injury, which can occur in all the conditions mentioned except tuberculosis. Indeed, the alveoli-lining, fibrinlike material may be found in multiple conditions of circulatory compromise and in poor perfusion states, such as hypovolemia; it may also be seen where 100% oxygen has been used for longer than 32 h (e.g., "shock lung" of Vietnam casualties). At autopsy, the lungs are relatively airless and heavy, and this finding is frequently accompanied by pulmonary edema and hemorrhage.

238–241. The answers are: 238-D, 239-A, 240-E, 241-C. *(Anderson, 9/e. p 1013. Robbins, 4/e. pp 574, 794.)* Oat cell carcinomas, which are of neuroendocrine origin and display neurosecretory granules on electron microscopy, may cause a variety of syndromes, some from direct synthesis of hormones such as ACTH and serotonin. Other effects, not well understood, on the neuromuscular system include central encephalopathy and Eaton-Lambert syndrome, a myasthenic syndrome resulting from impaired release of acetylcholine and usually associated with pulmonary oat cell carcinoma. Oat cell carcinomas form 20 to 25 percent of primary lung tumors, occur most frequently in middle-aged or older men, have a strong association with cigarette smoking, and carry a poor prognosis.

Both Wegener's granulomatosis, a syndrome of necrotizing vasculitis with necrotizing granulomas of nasopharynx and lung, and Goodpasture's syndrome, a disease produced by autoantibodies directed against basement membranes, typically involve both the lung and kidney. Goodpasture's syndrome is characterized by development of a necrotizing hemorrhagic interstitial pneumonitis and rapidly progressing glomerulonephritis because of antibodies directed against the capillary basement membrane in alveolar septae and glomeruli. Prognosis for Goodpasture's syndrome has been markedly improved by intensive plasma exchange to remove circulating antibasement membrane antibodies and by immunosuppressive therapy to inhibit further antibody production. In Wegener's granulomatosis, the nose, sinus, antrum, and trachea often exhibit ulcerations. Originally lethal, prognosis is now much improved by immunosuppressive drugs.

Byssinosis, which is caused by inhalation of cotton, flax, or hemp dust, takes the form of an asthmatic bronchitis, rather than involving distal lung structures, as with other organic dusts that cause extrinsic allergic alveolitis. Prolonged exposure causes chronic lung disease with chronic bronchitis, emphysema, and interstitial granulomas.

242–244. The answers are: 242-B, 243-D, 244-C. *(Anderson, 9/e. p 1017. Robbins, 4/e. pp 800, 802–803, 814–815.)* Bronchial carcinoids form about 5 percent of lung tumors. Sex incidence is equal and many patients are under 40 years of age. No relation to cigarette smoking or environmental factors is known. The origin is the neuroendocrine argentaffin cells of bronchial mucosa (Kultschitzsky cells). The carcinoid syndrome (diarrhea, facial flushing, and cyanosis) rarely occurs in disease confined to the lung. Carcinoid belongs to the group of amine precursor uptake and decarboxylation (APUD) tumors.

Bronchioloalveolar carcinoma, a form of adenocarcinoma, arises from terminal bronchioles and extends to line alveolar spaces throughout peripheral lung tissue, often causing a pneumonia-like picture grossly and radiologically. Ultrastructurally it consists of mucin-secreting bronchiolar cells, Clara cells, and, rarely, type II pneumocytes.

Adenoid cystic carcinoma may arise at any level of the respiratory tract where there are mucous glands and is the most common tumor in the upper third of the trachea. Histopathologic appearance is similar to adenoid cystic carcinoma of minor salivary glands with a cribriform, lacelike pattern of either duct-lining secretory cells or myoepithelial cells. Pools of mucoid material are actually extracellular matrix.

Nasopharyngeal angiofibroma is a highly vascular tumor that can cause heavy bleeding and occurs in young males. Other rare, but distinctive nasal tumors include isolated plasmacytoma, lymphoepithelioma, olfactory neuroblastoma (esthesioneuroblastoma), inverted papilloma, and carcinomas of epidermoid and transitional cell types.

245–248. The answers are: 245-E, 246-D, 247-A, 248-B. (*Wilson, 12/e. pp 557–558, 634–637, 746–747, 752–753.*) Legionnaire's disease is caused by the soil organism *Legionella pneumophila,* a weakly gram-negative aerobic bacillus (Legionellaceae, of over 25 species). The disease results from inhalation of infectious aerosols from hot water or air-conditioning systems of buildings (including hospitals); these aerosols contain legionellae, which are deposited in the lung alveoli. Legionellosis ranges from the fulminant pneumonia of Legionnaire's disease (first recognized in Philadelphia, 1976) to the mild, flulike Pontiac fever. Diarrhea, nausea, and vomiting are early symptoms as well as headache, fever, and often delirium. Gastrointestinal symptoms, briefly preceding pneumonia and scant (later mucoid) sputum, should suggest a diagnosis of Legionnaire's disease. Chest x-ray shows dense infiltrates with pulmonary gross findings of a confluent bronchopneumonia with alveoli containing neutrophils and mononuclear phagocytes with many intracytoplasmic bacilli that may be seen by silver staining. Organisms are also detected by immunofluorescent staining and culture of lung tissue, pleural fluid, or transtracheal aspirate, but not sputum culture since other organisms overgrow legionellae. Direct fluorescent antibody staining is specific, but relatively insensitive compared with lung biopsy culture or tracheal aspirate culture. Erythromycin is the favored therapy.

Nocardia (Nocardia asteroides) and *Actinomyces* are classified as filamentous soil bacteria, although they are often described among the fungi.

Nocardiae are aerobic and acid-fast in contrast to *Actinomyces,* which are strict anaerobes and not acid-fast. Inhaled nocardial bacteria produce lung or skin infections; progressive pneumonia with purulent sputum and abscesses is suggestive of nocardiosis, especially if dissemination to brain or subcutaneous tissue occurs. Patients developing nocardiosis are often immunosuppressed, and transplant rejection, steroid therapy, AIDS, and alveolar proteinosis are often antecedent. Organisms in sputum, pus, or bronchial lavage specimens are gram-positive and show beaded, refractile hyphae branching at right angles. A modified acid-fast stain should be used. Actinomycosis has cervicofacial, abdominal, thoracic, and pelvic (some IUD use) forms and occurs in normal hosts, though trauma and devitalized tissues play a part. Both *Nocardia* and *Actinomyces* cause abscesses and the actinomycotic abscess contains yellow bacterial colonies ("sulfur granules"). *Nocardia* and *Actinomyces* both belong to the order Actinomycetales.

Coccidioidomycosis, caused by inhalation of *C. immitis* arthrospores from airborne dust, is prevalent in California (San Joaquin Valley), Arizona, West Texas, and New Mexico. It may present clinically with hypersensitivity reactions—erythema nodosum or multiforme plus arthralgias and arthritis (desert rheumatism). These reactions are more frequent with coccidioidomycosis than with other mycoses. Pulmonary infection with infiltrate, hilar adenopathy, or pleural effusion is prominent and may become chronic and progressive with dissemination to bone, skin, and meninges. This occurs in less than 1 percent of cases. Diagnosis is by finding organisms in sputum or pus, but confirmation by direct immunofluorescence or culture may be necessary. Serologic tests are valuable in establishing diagnosis, and with the reactive antibodies, precipitin, latex agglutination, or immunodiffusion, tests are positive in most symptomatic cases. Complement-fixing antibodies in the CSF are diagnostic of meningitis. Many cases of *Coccidioides* infection are asymptomatic. When present, dermal hypersensitivity is a good prognostic sign.

Factors that contribute to staphylococcal pathogenicity include production of coagulase, catalase, enterotoxin, and exotoxin. Some strains of coagulase-positive staphylococci *(S. aureus)* produce exotoxins that cause skin lesions (scalded skin syndrome) or multisystem dysfunction, as in toxic shock syndrome in which rash, fever, and hypotension are present. Coagulase and catalase help to protect staphylococci from destruction by phagocytosis. Some strains produce an enterotoxin that causes gastrointestinal disease.

Type 3 pneumococcal infection has a higher mortality than that of other pneumococcal types, probably because type 3 often occurs in the aged or debilitated. Lung abscess is more likely to follow infection with pneumococcus type 3. Diseases produced by different pneumococcal serotypes show little variation in severity, apart from the higher mortality with type 3.

Gastrointestinal System

DIRECTIONS: Each question below contains five suggested responses. Select the **one best** response to each question.

249. The photomicrograph below shows the colonic wall 30 cm from the anal margin in a man with severe bloody diarrhea. All the statements regarding this condition are true EXCEPT

(A) inflammation is usually limited to the lamina propria
(B) multiple crypt abscesses are commonly seen
(C) atypical cytologic changes occur in the mucosa
(D) granulomas occur in the mucosa
(E) endarteritis obliterans occurs in the submucosal arteries

250. A 25-year-old schoolteacher was well until she attended a church bazaar where she heartily ate barbecued turkey. The following day she developed bloody diarrhea, crampy pain, and tenesmus. A gastroenterologist who did not take a history took a colon biopsy specimen that showed mucosal edema, congestion, and numerous lymphoid cells in the lamina propria. Which of the following differential diagnoses would apply?

(A) Staphylococcal gastroenteritis vs. Crohn's disease
(B) Viral gastroenteritis vs. acute diverticulitis
(C) Colonic endometriosis vs. amebic dysentery
(D) Early ulcerative colitis vs. *Salmonella* colitis
(E) Bleeding hemorrhoids vs. Meckel's diverticulitis

251. The photomicrograph below shows a section through the gallbladder wall. Which of the following statements regarding the condition illustrated is true?

(A) It is known as cholesterolosis
(B) Changes often extend into the extrahepatic bile ducts
(C) It predisposes to acute cholecystitis
(D) It is strongly associated with pigment stones
(E) None of the above

252. A 32-year-old woman sees her physician because of "stiffness" and intolerance to cold temperatures in her fingers. Her face has a "mask-like" quality. It would be appropriate in the systems review to ask about

(A) headaches and dizziness
(B) swallowing difficulties
(C) sun hypersensitivity
(D) thyroid trouble
(E) family history

253. The lesion seen in the photomicrograph below is referred to as

(A) adenoid cystic carcinoma
(B) lymphoepithelioma
(C) thyroglossal duct neoplasm
(D) Warthin's tumor
(E) sebaceous lymphadenoma

254. Which of the following statements regarding transmural intestinal infarction is true?

(A) Thromboemboli usually originate in the ileofemoral veins
(B) The colon is more commonly affected than the small intestine
(C) Colonic infarction classically affects the hepatic flexure
(D) Arterial occlusion results in pallor of the affected segment
(E) Up to 25 percent of cases are due to nonocclusive hypoperfusion

255. Gastric tumors with the histologic appearance illustrated in the photomicrograph below

(A) usually fall into the category of early gastric carcinoma
(B) are most commonly located in the cardia
(C) often show a marked desmoplastic response
(D) carry a favorable prognosis
(E) belong to the category of neuroendocrine tumors

256. Finely nodular (micronodular) cirrhosis, as illustrated in the photomicrograph below, is seen in all the following conditions EXCEPT

(A) postnecrotic cirrhosis
(B) secondary biliary cirrhosis
(C) primary biliary cirrhosis
(D) alcoholic cirrhosis
(E) hemochromatosis

257. The abnormality of the ileum illustrated below

(A) is present in approximately 10 percent of normal persons
(B) is lined by specialized gastric mucosa in the majority of cases
(C) often shows mucosal ulceration
(D) may be the site of a primary carcinoid tumor
(E) usually arises from the mesenteric border of the ileum

258. All the following statements concerning carcinoma of the stomach are true EXCEPT

(A) diffusely infiltrative carcinoma is associated with a striking desmoplastic reaction
(B) *early gastric carcinoma (EGC)* is synonymous with *carcinoma in situ*
(C) over 50 percent of gastric carcinomas are found in the pylorus and antrum
(D) there is a striking geographic variation in death rate from gastric carcinoma
(E) the death rate from gastric carcinoma has been decreasing for decades

259. The photomicrograph below was prepared after a distal colonic biopsy was performed. The most likely diagnosis is

(A) clonorchiasis
(B) enterobiasis
(C) filariasis
(D) strongyloidiasis
(E) schistosomiasis

260. All the following statements regarding carcinoma of the esophagus are true EXCEPT

(A) most carcinomas arising in the body of the esophagus are squamous
(B) squamous carcinomas begin as lesions in situ
(C) patients with Barrett's esophagus have approximately a 10 percent risk of carcinoma
(D) the most common morphologic form is a polypoid fungating mass
(E) distant metastases are frequently present at the time of diagnosis

261. In the photograph below, an ulcerated mucosal lesion is shown at the anorectal junction. This lesion is

(A) a villous adenoma
(B) a basaloid carcinoma
(C) a hemorrhoid
(D) a polypoid adenoma
(E) a mesenteric thrombus

262. The photomicrograph below shows an esophageal biopsy taken 10 cm above the lower esophageal sphincter. The condition illustrated

(A) is usually congenital in origin
(B) results from loss of esophageal myenteric ganglion cells
(C) is seen as a white patch at endoscopy
(D) increases the risk of carcinoma by a factor of 30 to 40
(E) is a common precursor of squamous cell carcinoma

263. Familial polyposis coli is characterized by

(A) autosomal recessive pattern of inheritance
(B) multiple hamartomatous polyps throughout the colon
(C) 100 percent risk of carcinoma within 30 years of diagnosis
(D) an association with fibromatosis and multiple osteomas
(E) an association with tumors of the central nervous system

264. A mononuclear portal inflammatory infiltrate that disrupts the limiting plate and surrounds individual hepatocytes (piecemeal necrosis), as shown in the photomicrograph below, is characteristic of

(A) ascending cholangitis
(B) chronic active hepatitis
(C) acute alcoholic hepatitis
(D) cholestatic jaundice
(E) nutritional cirrhosis

265. A middle-aged patient is undergoing surgical exploration for a tumor in the pancreatic fundus. No clinical history is given to the pathologist, who notes that the tumor has an "endocrine" appearance in frozen section. An appropriate step in the subsequent evaluation would be to consider

(A) immunoperoxidase
(B) brain scans
(C) computerized tomography
(D) celiac angiography
(E) immunofluorescence testing

266. The appearances of the small intestinal mucosa illustrated in the photo-micrograph below are those of

(A) small intestinal lymphoma
(B) Whipple's disease
(C) celiac disease
(D) Crohn's disease
(E) *Giardia lamblia* infestation

267. All the following statements concerning carcinoma of the colo-rectum are true EXCEPT

(A) 95 percent of all carcinomas of the colorectum are adenocarci-noma
(B) mucin secretion aids extension of the primary malignancy
(C) left-sided lesions tend to grow as polypoid fungating masses
(D) serum levels of carcinoem-bryonic antigen (CEA) are di-rectly related to size and spread
(E) serum levels of CEA fall to zero with complete removal of the tumor

268. A middle-aged male alcoholic has had repeated bouts of pancreatitis following periods of binge drinking. In recent months he has had a low-grade fever, and on examination a mass is palpated in the epigastrium. This mass, removed at celicotomy, is shown in the photograph below. What is the diagnosis?

(A) Pancreatic carcinoma
(B) Mucinous cystadenoma
(C) Perforated ulcer
(D) Pancreatic pseudocyst
(E) Cystic hepatoma

269. Tumors of the salivary glands are correctly characterized by which of the following statements?
(A) They are principally mesenchymal in origin
(B) They metastasize early and pursue a rapid course when malignant
(C) They tend to present similarly regardless of histologic pattern
(D) They are less often malignant in the minor salivary glands than in the parotid
(E) None of the above

270. The lesion shown in the colon in the photograph below

(A) is most prevalent under 50 years of age
(B) occurs most often in the ascending and transverse segments when it occurs in the colon
(C) occurs more often in the small intestine than the colon
(D) is more common in males
(E) is premalignant

271. Which of the following statements regarding alcoholic steatosis and hepatitis as illustrated in the photomicrograph below is true?

(A) Morphologic changes of steatosis are irreversible
(B) Hepatocyte necrosis is most marked in the periportal area
(C) Perivenular and pericellular fibroses are precursors of cirrhosis
(D) Mallory's hyaline is pathognomonic of alcoholic liver damage
(E) The inflammatory infiltrate is chiefly lymphocytic

272. A 65-year-old man presents with episodes of facial flushing exacerbated by alcohol and associated with severe diarrhea. All the following findings may be expected on further investigation EXCEPT

(A) increased urinary levels of 5-hydroxyindoleacetic acid (5-HIAA)
(B) elevated levels of serotonin in circulating platelets
(C) areas of decreased uptake on liver scintillation scan
(D) right-sided cardiac failure
(E) a small yellow nodule in the tip of the appendix

273. Two subtotal colectomy specimens are sent to the laboratory with both showing a hemorrhagic cobblestone appearance of the mucosa. One, however, shows longitudinal grooving of the surface, which suggests

(A) ischemic bowel disease
(B) multiple polyposis syndrome
(C) ulcerative colitis
(D) Crohn's disease
(E) none of the above

274. All the following statements regarding *Helicobacter pylori* gastritis as illustrated in the photomicrograph below are true EXCEPT

(A) it is present in the majority of patients with duodenal ulceration
(B) the inflammatory infiltrate is characteristically rich in eosinophils
(C) tissue invasion by microorganisms is inconspicuous
(D) organisms are absent from areas of intestinal metaplasia
(E) urease is an important virulence factor of *H. pylori*

275. Which of the following statements regarding carcinoma of the
exocrine pancreas is true?

(A) It arises from secretory cells of
pancreatic acini
(B) It is decreasing in frequency
(C) It is most often located in the
tail of the pancreas
(D) It is more common in diabetics
than in nondiabetics
(E) It carries a 40 percent 5-year
survival

276. All the following statements regarding the condition illustrated below
are true EXCEPT

(A) over 95 percent of cases occur in the stomach or duodenum
(B) cases associated with Zollinger-Ellison syndrome are frequently atypi-
cal in location
(C) duodenal ulceration is associated with hypersecretion of acid
(D) gastric ulceration is associated with hypersecretion of acid
(E) size of gastric ulcer is not an accurate predictor of malignant potential

DIRECTIONS: Each group of questions below consists of four lettered headings followed by a set of numbered items. For each numbered item select

A	if the item is associated with	(A) **only**
B	if the item is associated with	(B) **only**
C	if the item is associated with	**both** (A) and (B)
D	if the item is associated with	**neither** (A) nor (B)

Each lettered heading may be used **once, more than once, or not at all.**

Questions 277–279

(A) Ulcerative colitis
(B) Crohn's disease
(C) Both
(D) Neither

277. Erythema nodosum

278. Crypt abscesses

279. Fibrinomucinous exudate

Questions 280–283

(A) Primary biliary cirrhosis
(B) Laennec's cirrhosis
(C) Both
(D) Neither

280. Alcohol abuse

281. Bile duct proliferation

282. Xanthomas of skin and ulcerative colitis

283. Equal sex incidence

DIRECTIONS: Each group of questions below consists of lettered headings followed by a set of numbered items. For each numbered item select the **one** lettered heading with which it is **most** closely associated. Each lettered heading may be used **once, more than once, or not at all.**

Questions 284–287

Match each of the clinical and pathologic patterns of malabsorption syndrome with the appropriate cause.

(A) Abetalipoproteinemia
(B) Primary intestinal lymphoma
(C) Whipple's disease
(D) Disaccharidase deficiency
(E) Systemic mastocytosis

284. Recent viral infection, persistent diarrhea, normal bowel mucosa

285. Arthralgias, lymphadenopathy, blunted villi distended by macrophages

286. Diarrhea unresponsive to gluten-free diet, blunted villi with chronic inflammatory infiltrate

287. Failure to thrive, steatorrhea, lipid vacuolation of mucosal cells

Questions 288–290

For each patient below choose the most appropriate biochemical or serologic test.

(A) Serum alpha-fetoprotein
(B) Anti-hepatitis B surface antigen antibody (anti-HBsAg)
(C) Antimitochondrial antibody (AMA)
(D) Antineutrophil cytoplasmic antibody (ANCA)
(E) Serum ferritin

288. A 52-year-old woman with pruritus and markedly elevated serum alkaline phosphatase

289. A 65-year-old man with cardiomegaly and insulin-dependent diabetes mellitus of recent onset

290. A 43-year-old man with esophageal varices and rapidly increasing ascites

Gastrointestinal System
Answers

249. The answer is D. *(Rosai, 7/e. pp 577–580.)* The condition illustrated is ulcerative colitis, an inflammatory disorder of unknown cause. It involves the distal colon with variable proximal extension. Grossly there is ulceration with islands of residual mucosa. The inflammation is predominantly superficial with an infiltrate of acute and chronic inflammatory cells in the lamina propria. Cryptitis and crypt abscesses are common. Many lymphoid follicles may be seen but epithelioid cells, giant cells, and granulomas are absent. Cellular atypia is seen in regenerating mucosa. Submucosal arteries show features of endarteritis obliterans in approximately 10 percent of cases. When ulcerative colitis is inactive, morphologic abnormalities of glands, goblet cell depletion, and Paneth cell metaplasia indicate underlying disease.

250. The answer is D. *(Robbins, 4/e. pp 353–355, 867–869, 886–889.)* Early stages of ulcerative colitis (UC) may be indistinguishable from gastroenteritis caused by *Salmonella choleraesuis* and *S. typhimurium*. In early stages, both diseases may show histologically a dense mononuclear inflammatory infiltrate in the lamina propria, occasional crypt abscesses, and mucosal edema and congestion. Even the respective clinical symptoms and colon x-ray changes may be similar, although marked vomiting should point to food poisoning. Salmonellae have been the cause of outbreaks and epidemics of acute gastroenteritis, and the cause has often been found to be contaminated fowl that has been insufficiently cooked to inactivate endotoxins.

251. The answer is A. *(Robbins, 4/e. pp 971–973.)* Cholesterolosis of the gallbladder, also known as "strawberry gallbladder," is relatively common and, although associated with cholesterol calculi, is not thought to predispose to acute cholecystitis or malignancy. Lipid-laden macrophages accumulate within the mucosal folds of the gallbladder and result in a yellow-flecked appearance. The pathophysiology is unclear but may be related to the presence of supersaturated bile. Following acute or chronic cholecystitis there may be diffuse calcium deposition in the gallbladder wall (calcified, or "porcelain," gallbladder), which is not associated with cholesterolosis. Pigment stones may occur with increased concentration of unconjugated bilirubin in bile, as in the hemolytic anemias.

252. The answer is B. (*Robbins, 4/e. pp 204–207, 579.*) The constellation of Raynaud's phenomenon, acral sclerosis, and fibrotic tightening of the muscles of facial expression should raise the specter of progressive systemic sclerosis (scleroderma), a multisystem disease that involves the cardiovascular, gastrointestinal, cutaneous, musculoskeletal, pulmonary, and renal systems through progressive interstitial fibrosis. Small arterioles in the forenamed systems show obliteration caused by intimal hyperplasia accompanied by progressive interstitial fibrosis. Evidence implicates a lymphocyte overdrive of fibroblasts to produce an excess of rather normal collagen. Eventually, myocardial fibrosis, pulmonary fibrosis, and terminal renal failure ensue. Over half of all patients have dysphagia with solid food caused by the distal esophageal narrowing in the disease.

253. The answer is D. (*Robbins, 4/e. pp 824–826.*) Warthin's tumors occur mainly in the lower regions of the parotid gland, especially near the angle of the mandible, and on rare occasion may be bilateral. They are completely benign neoplasms although they carry some undesirable synonyms: *adenolymphoma*, which is a misnomer, and *papillary cystadenoma lymphomatosum*, a term undesirable both for the *lymphomatosum* part as well as its length. For these reasons most workers prefer the term *Warthin's tumor.* The pattern is highly characteristic of an epithelial surface lining of acidophilic cells that overlay benign lymphoid tissue elements, including germinal centers. The epithelial portion probably arises from early duct cells that become entrapped within developing parotid lymph nodes during embryogenesis. Sebaceous lymphadenoma would have sebaceous cells within the lymphoid tissue. Thyroglossal duct cyst is located in the midline of the neck but may be found extending up to the base of the tongue, and there is a similarity between the lymphoid islands seen in thyroglossal duct cysts and in Warthin's tumor; however, thyroid follicles may lead to the correct diagnosis in the former. Lymphoepithelioma is a tumor that is recognized by hyperplastic duct epithelium surrounded by lymphoid tissue. Myoepithelial islands embedded in lymphoid tissue may be seen in the minor and major salivary glands in Sjögren's syndrome.

254. The answer is E. (*Robbins, 4/e. pp 863–864.*) Transmural intestinal infarction is that part of the spectrum of mesenteric ischemia in which there is ischemic necrosis of the full thickness of the intestinal wall. Fifty percent of cases involve the small intestine only and are a result of thrombotic or embolic occlusion of the superior mesenteric artery. Thromboemboli arise from intracardiac mural thrombi, prostheses or valvular vegetations, or from complicated atherosclerotic plaques in the aorta. Arterial thrombi usually occur over atherosclerotic plaques. Twenty-five percent of cases result from non-occlusive hypoperfusion of the small or large intestine.

Arterial and venous occlusion both lead to hemorrhagic infarction with intense congestion and discoloration of the affected bowel segment. The area of the colon most often affected is the splenic flexure, which represents the watershed region of supply between the superior and inferior mesenteric arteries.

255. The answer is C. *(Robbins, 4/e. pp 854–858.)* "Signet-ring cell" carcinoma is a morphologic variant of adenocarcinoma most often seen in the stomach. In these tumors, intracellular mucin vacuoles coalesce and distend the cytoplasm of tumor cells, which compresses the nucleus toward the edge of the cell and creates a "signet-ring" appearance. Tumors of this type are usually deeply invasive and fall into the category of advanced gastric carcinoma. There is often a striking desmoplasia with thickening and rigidity of the gastric wall, which may result in the so-called linitis plastica appearance. Advanced gastric carcinoma is usually located in the pyloroantrum and the prognosis is poor with 5-year survival of only 5 to 15 percent.

256. The answer is A. *(Robbins, 4/e. pp 941–956.)* Cirrhosis is often subdivided into micronodular and macronodular types on the basis of the size of individual nodules within the cirrhotic liver. Although this division is entirely descriptive, most diseases that lead to cirrhosis result in one of these subtypes. Alcoholic liver damage, hemochromatosis, and biliary cirrhosis typically result in a micronodular pattern with nodules < 3 mm in diameter. Postnecrotic cirrhosis is typically macronodular and a mixed or variable pattern may be seen in the cirrhosis of Wilson's disease and α_1-antitrypsin deficiency.

257. The answer is D. *(Rosai, 7/e. p 522.)* Meckel's diverticulum occurs in the ileum, usually within 80 cm of the ileocecal valve, and is present in approximately 2 percent of normal persons. It represents incomplete involution of the vitello-intestinal duct and always arises from the antimesenteric border of the intestine. Most cases are lined by small intestinal mucosa, but heterotopic gastric, colonic, or pancreatic tissue may be present. Peptic ulceration, which occurs as a result of acid secretion by heterotopic gastric mucosa, is usually located in the adjacent ileum. Complications include perforation, ulceration, intestinal obstruction, intussusception, and neoplasms, including carcinoid tumors.

258. The answer is B. *(Robbins, 4/e. pp 854–858.)* The death rate from gastric carcinoma has been decreasing for decades but still shows marked variations among countries; Japan, Chile, and Iceland have rates up to six times higher than those of the U.S. and Australia. First-generation migrants carry the risk of their country of origin, but subsequent generations assume the risk of their new country. *Early gastric carcinoma (EGC)* refers to a local neoplastic lesion limited to the mucosa and submucosa without penetration of the muscularis propria. Metastasis can occur, however, from EGC to local lymph nodes in up to 5 percent of cases. EGC is usually recognizable on radiographic or endoscopic examination, and so in most cases is potentially curable. It develops very slowly into a frankly invasive lesion and, if detected early and removed, allows a 5-year survival of up to 95 percent compared with 15 percent for gastric carcinoma overall. Of all gastric carcinomas, 50 to 60 percent arise in the pyloroantrum, 10 percent in the cardia, 10 percent in the whole organ, and the remainder in other sites. Diffusely infiltrative carcinoma extends widely through the stomach wall, often without producing an intraluminal mass, and incites a marked desmoplastic reaction that results in a thickened, inelastic stomach wall.

259. The answer is B. *(Anderson, 9/e. pp 464–465.)* In the photomicrograph, a cross section of an *Enterobius* adult worm is shown. Apparent morphologic features of this nematode include the bilateral crests, the meromyarial type of musculature, and the noncellular cuticle with spines. *Enterobius vermicularis,* the agent responsible for the helminthic infection most common in the United States, usually produces pruritus ani as the outstanding and most disturbing symptom of enterobiasis (pinworm infection). *Enterobius* worms often attach themselves to the cecal mucosa and contiguous regions, but the usual host sites for schistosomiasis, clonorchiasis, and filariasis are the veins of the large intestine, the bile ducts, and the lymphatics, respectively. Elephantiasis is a characteristic feature in filariasis, and infection by *Strongyloides stercoralis* usually produces hyperemia and edema of the mucosa of the small intestine.

260. The answer is E. *(Robbins, 4/e. pp 835–838.)* Carcinoma of the esophagus accounts for about 10 percent of malignancies of the GI tract, but for a disproportionate number of cancer deaths. Predisposing factors include smoking, esophagitis, and achalasia. Sixty to seventy percent are squamous cell carcinomas that characteristically begin as lesions in situ. Adenocarcinoma occurs mainly in the lower esophagus and may arise in up to 10 percent of cases of Barrett's esophagus. Anaplastic and small cell variants also occur. Polypoid lesions are most common, followed by malignant ulceration and diffusively infiltrative forms. Tumors tend to spread by direct invasion of adjacent structures, but lymphatic and hematogenous spread may occur. Distant metastases are, however, a late feature. Five-year survival is less than 10 percent.

261. The answer is B. *(Robbins, 4/e. p 902.)* The lesion pictured is a basaloid, or cloacogenic, carcinoma that has the same gross appearance as the more common epidermoid carcinoma, although the lesion histologically resembles the basal cell carcinoma of the skin. The tumor arises from the anal canal within the transitional zone epithelium (anal columns). Some of these tumors resemble transitional epithelium, whereas others vary in their patterns, including one pattern similar to that of small cell (oat cell) carcinoma of the lung and other patterns that are totally undifferentiated. The prognosis for cloacogenic carcinoma is directly proportional to the degree of differentiation.

262. The answer is D. *(Rosai, 7/e. pp 471–473.)* The presence of columnar epithelium lining part or all of the distal esophagus is known as *Barrett's esophagus*. It is considered an acquired change resulting from reflux of acidic gastric contents with ulceration of the esophageal squamous epithelium and replacement by metaplastic, acid-resistant, columnar epithelium. Endoscopically it has a velvety-red appearance. Microscopically, intestinal-type epithelium is most common, but gastric-type epithelium is also seen. Varying degrees of dysplasia may be present. The risk of carcinoma is increased 30- to 40-fold. Virtually all of these tumors are of adenocarcinoma type and they account for up to 10 percent of all esophageal cancers.

263. The answer is C. *(Robbins, 4/e. pp 896–897.)* Although most colonic polyps occur sporadically, there are several conditions in which colonic polyposis is familial and sometimes associated with extraintestinal abnormalities. Familial polyposis coli is usually transmitted as an autosomal dominant condition and is characterized by multiple adenomatous colonic polyps with a minimum of 100 polyps necessary for diagnosis. As with sporadic adenomatous polyps, there is a risk of malignancy and this increases to 100 percent within 30 years of diagnosis. Panproctocolectomy is, therefore, usually recommended. Gardner's syndrome is the association of colonic polyposis with multiple osteomas, fibromatosis, and cutaneous cysts. The association of colonic polyposis with central nervous system tumors is known as Turcot's syndrome.

264. The answer is B. *(Robbins, 4/e. pp 924–937.)* Chronic hepatitis has been defined as an inflammatory process of the liver that lasts longer than 1 year and lacks the nodular regeneration and architectural distortion of cirrhosis. In chronic active hepatitis, an intense inflammatory reaction with numerous plasma cells spreads from portal tracts into periportal areas. The reaction destroys the limiting plate and results in formation of periportal hepatocytic islets. Prognosis is poor, and the majority of patients develop cirrhosis. Chronic persistent hepatitis is usually a sequela of acute viral hepatitis and has a benign course, without progression to chronic active hepatitis or cirrhosis. The portal inflammation does not extend into the periportal areas, and this differentiates it from chronic active hepatitis.

265. The answer is A. *(Robbins, 4/e. pp 1005–1008. Schwarz, N Engl J Med 305:917, 1981.)* Any tumor of the pancreas seen to have an organoid (endocrine-like) pattern histologically, even in frozen section, should arouse suspicion of an islet cell tumor, a carcinoid, or a component tumor of multiple endocrine neoplasia. The pathologist may be alert to this possibility if appropriate clinical information relating the patient's symptoms accompanies the biopsy specimen. Electron microscopy will show specialized types of electron-dense core granules ("neurosecretory" granules) in the cytoplasm in the presence of tumors of the amine precursor uptake decarboxylation class (APUDomas). Islet cell tumors may contain alpha (glucagon), beta (insulin), delta (somatostatin), and pp (pancreatic polypeptide) dense-core granules. Direct staining of the hormones can be accomplished with immunoperoxidase, which contains the specific antibody to the hormone being sought and forms rust-brown granules that can be seen with the ordinary light microscope.

266. The answer is C. *(Robbins, 4/e. pp 876–877.)* Celiac disease, or gluten-sensitive enteropathy, is an inflammatory condition of the small intestinal mucosa related to dietary gluten. It is more common in females and shows familial clustering. Histologically it is characterized by loss of villous architecture (villus atrophy) with hyperplasia of underlying crypts and increased mitotic activity. The surface epithelium shows disarray of the columnar epithelial cells and increased intraepithelial lymphocytes. There is a chronic inflammatory infiltrate in the lamina propria. Definitive diagnosis in patients with these features on biopsy depends on response to a gluten-free diet and subsequent gluten challenge.

267. The answer is C. *(Robbins, 4/e. pp 897–901.)* Ninety-five percent of all carcinomas of the colorectum are adenocarcinoma. The remainder are adenosquamous or adenoacanthoma. Many of the adenocarcinomas secrete mucin. When this secretion is extracellular, it dissects the gut wall cell planes and so aids extension of the malignancy. The gross pathology of left- and right-sided lesions differs; left-sided lesions tend to grow in an annular encircling fashion, while right-sided lesions tend to be sessile or polypoid fungating masses. Carcinoembryonic antigen is the tumor marker longest used in diagnosis and follow-up of colorectal tumors. Its serum levels are directly related to both size and extent of spread of the primary tumor. With large neoplasms there is almost 100 percent positivity. Levels fall to zero with complete removal of tumor but rise again with recurrence at primary or secondary sites.

268. The answer is D. *(Robbins, 4/e. pp 988–989.)* Pseudocysts of the pancreas are so named because the cystic structure is essentially unlined by any type of epithelium. True cysts, wherever they are found in the body, are always lined by some type of epithelium, whether columnar cell, glandular, squamous, or flattened cuboidal cell. The pancreatic pseudocyst is most commonly found in a background of repeated episodes of pancreatitis. Eventual mechanical large duct obstruction by either an inflammatory process per se, periductal fibrosis, or an abscess along with inspissated duct fluid from secretions and enzymes leads to the expanding mass. The mass lesion may be located between the stomach and liver, between the stomach and colon or transverse mesocolon, or in the lesser sac. Drainage or excision is necessary for adequate treatment. Acute bacterial infection may complicate the course.

269. The answer is C. *(Robbins, 4/e. pp 822–826.)* The salivary glands give rise to a wide variety of tumors, the majority of which are of epithelial origin and benign. Approximately 75 to 85 percent occur in the parotids, 10 to 20 percent in the submandibular glands, and the remainder in the minor glands. In the parotid the vast majority are benign, whereas in the minor glands 35 to 50 percent are malignant. Mesenchymal tumors are rare. Clinically, most tumors of salivary glands present as palpable masses, regardless of histologic type. They occasionally present with symptoms related to local invasion, such as facial nerve palsy. Masses may be present for years before diagnosis, even when malignant. Carcinomas tend to run an indolent course, invade local structures slowly, recur locally after removal, and metastasize late. Prognosis is usually presented in 10- or 20-year survival rates.

270. The answer is D. *(Anderson, 9/e. p 1155.)* Diverticula occur most frequently in men over the age of 50 and are most often located in the descending and sigmoid colon. The colon is the most commonly involved segment of the gastrointestinal tract. A majority of these lesions are not true diverticula since the mucosa and muscularis mucosae herniate through defects in the muscularis propria. Complications are not very common but include diverticulitis, hemorrhage, perforation, fistulas, intestinal obstruction, and, more commonly, bowel spasms or abnormal motility (irritable bowel syndrome).

271. The answer is C. *(Robbins, 4/e. pp 944–949.)* Alcoholic liver disease includes steatosis (fatty liver), hepatitis, and cirrhosis. Steatosis is the earliest hepatic consequence of excess alcohol intake and consists of cytoplasmic accumulation of lipid vacuoles that coalesce and distend the cells with ultrastructural evidence of cell injury. These changes are reversible. Alcoholic hepatitis is usually accompanied by some fatty changes and is characterized by hepatocellular swelling, necrosis, and neutrophil infiltration in the perivenular area, as well as the appearance of Mallory's hyaline—eosinophilic cytoplasmic inclusions composed of cytokeratin proteins. These inclusions may also, however, be seen in liver injury due to other causes. Pericellular fibrosis and fibrosis around the central vein are significant changes considered by some to indicate the possible development of cirrhosis.

272. The answer is E. *(Robbins, 4/e. pp 872–875.)* The patient shows two of the most common clinical manifestations of the carcinoid syndrome. Flushing is found in 90 percent, diarrhea in 75 percent, bronchoconstriction in 20 percent, and right-sided endocardial fibrosis in 35 percent of patients with the carcinoid syndrome. The syndrome results from elaboration of serotonin by a primary carcinoid tumor in the lungs or ovary, or from hepatic metastases from a primary carcinoid tumor in the gastrointestinal tract. Diagnosis is based on finding increased urinary 5-HIAA excretion from metabolism of excess serotonin and on histologic analysis of tumor tissue. Primary appendiceal carcinoid tumors very rarely metastasize and are virtually always asymptomatic.

273. The answer is D. *(Robbins, 4/e. pp 868–872.)* Hemorrhagic cobblestone appearance of the colon and small bowel may be seen in multiple states including inflammatory bowel disease, a term that can apply both to ulcerative colitis and regional enteritis (Crohn's disease). Other conditions that resemble cobblestoning of the mucosa of the bowel include multiple polyps such as occur in Gardner's syndrome, Turcot syndrome, familial polyposis, and multiple acquired polyps. Crohn's disease, however, differs from the others in that longitudinal ulcers may be present, yielding a long axis grooving, parallel to the long axis of the bowel. Such ulcers may also be seen in tuberculous enteritis; however, when inflammatory bowel disease is in the differential diagnosis, longitudinal ulcers are indicative of Crohn's disease.

274. The answer is B. *(Peterson, N Engl J Med 324:1043–1048, 1991. Robbins, 4/e. pp 845–847.)* Helicobacter pylori is a gram-negative, microaerophilic, curved bacillus found only on gastric-type epithelium. It is present in 10 percent of normal persons under 30 years of age with prevalence rising to 60 percent in those over 60 years of age. Virtually all patients with duodenal ulceration and 80 percent of those with gastric ulceration are infected by *H. pylori*. Many virulence factors aid the organism in colonization of the acid environment of the stomach, one of the most important of which is urease, which produces ammonia and buffers gastric acidity. The organism does not invade the tissues but induces surface epithelial cell damage and an inflammatory infiltrate in the lamina propria that is typically superficial and mixed granulocytic and lymphocytic.

275. The answer is D. *(Robbins, 4/e. pp 990–992.)* Carcinoma of the exocrine pancreas is a highly malignant tumor that accounts for 5 percent of cancer deaths in the U.S. Its occurrence has increased threefold in the past 40 years mainly as a result of smoking and exposure to chemical carcinogens. It is more frequent in diabetics than nondiabetics. Sixty percent of tumors are located in the head of the pancreas, 20 percent in the body, and 5 percent in the tail. The remainder are of indeterminate primary location. Growth is often insidious and presentation is often with jaundice due to compression of the extrahepatic bile ducts. The disease is rarely curable at presentation and prognosis is poor, with median survival from diagnosis of 6 months and 5-year survival of only 1 to 2 percent.

276. The answer is D. *(Robbins, 4/e. pp 850–852, 1007.)* Peptic ulceration may occur anywhere in the gastrointestinal tract exposed to acid-peptic activity. Over 98 percent of cases occur in the stomach or duodenum with duodenal outnumbering gastric by 4:1. Ulcers associated with the Zollinger-Ellison syndrome are typically multiple and frequently involve distal duodenum and jejunum. Differences exist in the pathogenesis of ulceration in the stomach and duodenum: duodenal ulceration appears to be related to hypersecretion of acid and to *H. pylori* infection; gastric ulceration typically occurs in a setting of normo- or hypochlorhydria with abnormality of mucosal defense mechanisms, back-diffusion of acid, and possibly local ischemia. Peptic ulcers are usually small but up to 10 percent of benign gastric ulcers are > 4 cm in diameter; malignant ulcers may be small.

277–279. The answers are: 277-C, 278-A, 279-D. *(Robbins, 4/e. pp 869–871, 887–889.)* Ulcerative colitis and Crohn's disease may show very similar morphologic features. Useful findings in distinguishing the two include total colonic involvement, distal predominance, broad-based ulcers, pseudopolyps, and crypt abscesses, all of which are more frequently found in ulcerative colitis; and skip lesions, serpentine fissures, transmural inflammation, lymphoid aggregates, granulomas, and fibrous thickening, which suggest a diagnosis of Crohn's disease. Extragastrointestinal manifestations such as erythema nodosum, arthritis, uveitis, pericholangitis, and ankylosing spondylitis may be associated with both ulcerative colitis and Crohn's disease. Fissures and cutaneous fistulas in the perineum are suggestive of Crohn's disease, rather than ulcerative colitis.

A fibrinomucinous exudate that appears to erupt from the mucosal crypts and is associated with a normal or hyperemic mucosa is found in pseudomembranous colitis (PMC). PMC is usually caused by the toxin of *Clostridium difficile,* although it may also result from infection by staphylococcus, shigella, or candida, or from ischemia. Most often it occurs after broad-spectrum antibiotics—such as clindamycin, lincomycin, or ampicillin—have been given.

280–283. The answers are: 280-B, 281-C, 282-A, 283-D. *(Anderson, 9/e. pp 1208–1210, 1244–1247, 1254–1257.)* Alcohol abuse, alcoholic hepatitis, and Laennec's (micronodular) cirrhosis are closely related. Cirrhosis of alcoholic liver disease is characterized by micronodules of regenerated hepatocytes surrounded by peripheral fibrosis. Central veins are only rarely seen within the pseudonodules. The fibrotic network contains varying bile duct proliferation and chronic inflammatory cells.

Atypical bile duct proliferation is a diagnostic feature of primary biliary cirrhosis (PBC), although it also occurs in Laennec's cirrhosis. High levels of serum cholesterol result in dermal xanthomas and ulcerative colitis and are associated with PBC. PBC presents in middle-aged women, who experience pruritus, jaundice, and nontender hepatomegaly. Alkaline phosphatase levels in the serum are elevated, and antimitochondrial antibodies can be demonstrated. There is evidence that PBC is autoimmune, with sensitized T cells involved in the granulomatous and bile duct inflammatory lesions. There is a gradual loss of intrahepatic bile ducts after an initial stage of lymphocytic and granulomatous inflammation. This is followed by a stage of bile duct proliferation. The third stage is active fibrosis.

Laennec's cirrhosis occurs more frequently in men. Primary biliary cirrhosis occurs much more frequently in women (9:1 ratio).

284–287. The answers are: 284-D, 285-C, 286-B, 287-A. *(Robbins, 4/e. pp 875–881. Wilson, 12/e. pp 1256–1263.)* Malabsorption syndromes have protean causes and are broadly categorized on the basis of the underlying abnormality. Abetalipoproteinemia is a rare condition in which absence of lipoprotein B leads to inability to synthesize prebetalipoproteins (VLDL), betalipoproteins (LDL), and chylomicrons. Consequently, lipid accumulates in vacuoles in mucosal cells.

Whipple's disease is a multisystem disorder of presumed infectious origin. The lamina propria of the small intestinal mucosa is distended by PAS-positive macrophages containing bacillary bodies. The condition usually responds to broad-spectrum antibiotics.

Primary intestinal lymphoma usually arises in men under the age of 50 and may present with malabsorption. Malignant lymphoid cells infiltrate the lamina propria of the mucosa. Lymphadenopathy and hepatosplenomegaly are usually absent.

Disaccharidase (usually lactase) deficiency is most commonly secondary to infection, inflammation, celiac disease, or radiation enteritis; it is rarely inherited. Lactose cannot be broken down and the resulting osmotic load causes diarrhea. Morphology is normal and diagnosis is based on lactose challenge.

288–290. The answers are: 288-C, 289-E, 290-A. *(Robbins, 4/e. pp 950–954, 959–962. Wilson, 12/e. pp 1343–1344.)* Primary biliary cirrhosis (PBC) is an idiopathic cholestatic condition that leads to cirrhosis. It is nine times more frequent in females and the average age of onset is 50 to 55 years. It is often insidious in onset, many patients being asymptomatic or with only pruritus despite a markedly increased serum alkaline phosphatase. Various autoantibodies may be present in the serum but the most sensitive and specific is antimitochondrial antibody, which is present in more than 90 percent of symptomatic patients. Diagnosis should be confirmed by liver biopsy.

Primary hemochromatosis is a genetic disorder that affects men five times more frequently than women. In this disease excessive amounts of iron are deposited in the parenchymal cells of various organs. Total body iron stores are grossly elevated. The organs chiefly affected are the liver, pancreas, myocardium, and endocrine glands; this may lead to cirrhosis, cardiomegaly and cardiac failure, and diabetes mellitus. In established cases serum iron is often >250 µg/dL and serum ferritin >500 ng/dL.

Primary hepatocellular carcinoma represents 2 to 3 percent of all malignant neoplasms in the Western world and arises on a background of cirrhosis in 80 to 95 percent of these cases. Clinical presentation is often nonspecific, but hepatomegaly and ascites are usually present. Alpha$_1$-antitrypsin and alpha-fetoprotein may be demonstrated in the tumor cells by immunocytochemistry in up to 75 percent of cases, and 75 percent of cases also show elevated serum levels of alpha-fetoprotein, which is not seen in cirrhosis alone.

Endocrine System

DIRECTIONS: Each question below contains five suggested responses. Select the **one best** response to each question.

291. The most common etiologic factor in Cushing's syndrome is

(A) adrenal adenoma
(B) bilateral adrenal hyperplasia
(C) adrenal carcinoma
(D) ectopic adrenal tissue
(E) hypercorticism secondary to nonendocrine malignant tumors

292. An adult patient with seizure disorder controlled by phenytoin (Dilantin) is noted to have enlarged gingivae. Select the proper course of action below.

(A) No action is necessary because this is a drug effect
(B) No action is necessary because this is a physiologic response
(C) Schilling blood count should be performed
(D) Roentgenograms of the maxillae and mandible should be taken
(E) Biopsy with histologic examination should be performed

293. The combination of cystic bone lesions, precocious puberty, and patchy skin pigmentations is known as

(A) Albright's syndrome
(B) Letterer-Siwe disease
(C) Asherman's syndrome
(D) Morquio's disease
(E) Schaumann's disease

294. Follicular carcinoma of the thyroid may show all the following features EXCEPT

(A) vascular invasion and hematogenous metastasis
(B) multiple foci within the gland
(C) a clear cell variant that resembles renal carcinoma
(D) an insular type that is an aggressive form
(E) absence of ground-glass nuclei

295. Graves' disease is associated with all the following EXCEPT

(A) tachycardia
(B) anti-TSH receptor antibodies
(C) localized myxedema
(D) toxic nodular goiter
(E) exophthalmos

296. The section of tissue shown in the photomicrograph below (taken under low power) was probably removed from a patient who has

(A) a normal thyroid gland
(B) colloid storage goiter
(C) Graves' disease
(D) Riedel's struma
(E) Hashimoto's thyroiditis

297. All the following statements concerning thymomas are true EXCEPT

(A) they originate from epithelial cells
(B) they are most common in the anterosuperior mediastinum
(C) they are asymptomatic or cause local pressure effects
(D) neoplastic lymphocytes are a component
(E) most thymomas are benign

298. A 42-year-old man complains of recently having to change his shoe size from 9 to 10½, and he also says that his hands and jaw are now larger. The disorder is most likely mediated through

(A) prolactin
(B) ACTH
(C) somatomedin
(D) antidiuretic hormone
(E) thyrotropin

299. A perimenopausal woman complains of slight swallowing difficulty, fatigue, and a change in bowel habits. The photomicrograph below is of her thyroid gland. This disorder is

(A) subacute thyroiditis
(B) thyrotoxicosis
(C) autoimmune thyroiditis
(D) Riedel's thyroiditis
(E) conversion hysteria

---

300. Myelolipoma of the adrenal displays all the following characteristics EXCEPT

(A) origination in the inner zona fasciculata
(B) average diameter of 0.5 to 6 cm
(C) occasional intercostal and retroperitoneal occurrence
(D) rare inclusion of adrenocortical cells
(E) rare and late metastases

301. Primary hyperaldosteronism is associated with all the following features EXCEPT

(A) carcinoma
(B) adenoma
(C) muscle weakness
(D) expansion of intravascular volume
(E) edema

Questions 302–303

302. A young patient with renal insufficiency and bone lesions undergoes surgical neck exploration for investigation of a metabolic defect. The photomicrograph above indicates that the patient has

(A) malignant lymphoma
(B) chronic thyroiditis
(C) thyroid hyperplasia
(D) parathyroid hyperplasia
(E) Castelman's disease

303. These bone lesions represent

(A) lymphomatous dissemination
(B) osteomyelitis
(C) osteomalacia
(D) osteopetrosis
(E) osteochondrosis

304. The parathyroid glands can be described in terms of anatomic or developmental characteristics that include all the following EXCEPT

(A) embryonic development from the endodermal tissue of the third and fourth pharyngeal pouches
(B) the location of the superior glands normally at the lower border of the cricoid cartilage
(C) a spatial relationship with the thyroid and a temporal developmental relationship with the thymus
(D) usually four in number applied to the dorsum of the thyroid gland
(E) a constant location of the inferior glands

305. A 49-year-old man who smokes two packs of cigarettes a day presents with a lung mass on x-ray and recent weight gain. Laboratory examination shows hyponatremia with hyperosmolar urine. The patient probably has

(A) renal failure
(B) pituitary failure
(C) Conn's syndrome
(D) cardiac failure
(E) inappropriate ADH

DIRECTIONS: The group of questions below consists of four lettered headings followed by a set of numbered items. For each numbered item select

A	if the item is associated with	(A) **only**
B	if the item is associated with	(B) **only**
C	if the item is associated with	**both** (A) and (B)
D	if the item is associated with	**neither** (A) nor (B)

Each lettered heading may be used **once, more than once, or not at all.**

Questions 306–309

(A) Papillary carcinoma of the thyroid gland
(B) Medullary carcinoma of the thyroid gland
(C) Both
(D) Neither

306. Frequent follicular variants appear

307. Hematogenous metastasis is usual

308. Both sporadic and familial forms occur

309. Amyloid deposits are common

DIRECTIONS: Each group of questions below consists of lettered headings followed by a set of numbered items. For each numbered item select the **one** lettered heading with which it is **most** closely associated. Each lettered heading may be used **once, more than once, or not at all.**

Questions 310–313

For each disorder listed, select the most appropriate feature or description.

(A) Panhypopituitarism in adults
(B) Cushing's syndrome in childhood
(C) Rare condition with very rare elaboration of hormones
(D) Postpartum pituitary necrosis
(E) Common cause of diabetes insipidus in children

310. Hand-Schüller-Christian disease

311. Sheehan's syndrome

312. Simmonds' disease

313. Adrenal cortical carcinoma

Questions 314–317

For each endocrinopathy, select the most appropriate condition.

(A) Empty sella syndrome
(B) Tumor of adrenal medulla
(C) Bilateral adrenalectomy
(D) Most common endocrinopathy caused by pituitary tumor
(E) Excess secretion of hormone in chronic renal insufficiency

314. Secondary hyperparathyroidism

315. Multiple endocrine neoplasia (MEN type II)

316. Nelson's syndrome

317. Hyperprolactinemia

Endocrine System
Answers

291. The answer is B. *(Wilson, 12/e. pp 1720–1725.)* Cushing's syndrome may be the result of bilateral adrenal hyperplasia, adrenal neoplasia, or excessive use of adrenocorticotropic hormone or glucocorticoids. However, bilateral adrenal hyperplasia is the most common etiologic factor. The clinical manifestations of the syndrome—whether it is induced by ectopic ACTH (small cell carcinoma of the lung), or exogenously, or endogenously by the adrenal—are similar. Levels of plasma and urinary cortisol and urinary 17-hydroxycorticoid are usually elevated.

292. The answer is C. *(Robbins, 4/e. p 821.)* There are multiple causes for enlarged gingivae, some of which are physiologic and transient and require no investigative or therapeutic measures. Among these is pregnancy, which under the stimulation of hormones produces a vascular proliferation that presents histology similar to that of pyogenic granuloma. Another physiologic response is that seen at puberty. Nutritional disorders such as vitamin C deficiency can also lead to enlarged gums. Phenytoin (Dilantin) has been known to cause enlargement of the gums in some patients. If the setting does not suggest a physiologic response, consideration should be given to leukemia, especially monocytic leukemia, which can present enlarged gums as the initial manifestation. Thus, a complete blood count, including a Schilling differential to enumerate the white cells, is indicated.

293. The answer is A. *(Anderson, 9/e. pp 1898–1900.)* The triad of cystic bone lesions, precocious puberty, and patchy brownish skin pigmentation is known as Albright's syndrome. The bone lesions are those of fibrous dysplasia and apparently result from abnormal activity by the bone-forming mesenchyma. Packing of the medullary cavity by fibrous tissue that contains trabeculae of poorly mineralized fibrous bone is seen in the lesions. Recent reports have described cases of fibrous dysplasia in both males and females who also have had a wide variety of endocrine abnormalities, including hyperthyroidism, acromegaly, and Cushing's syndrome.

294. The answer is B. *(Robbins, 4/e. pp 1234–1238.)* The four major histologic subtypes of thyroid carcinoma, in decreasing order of frequency, are papillary, follicular, medullary, and undifferentiated (anaplastic). Follicular carcinoma has a frequency of approximately 10 to 20 percent compared with papillary cancer at 60 to 70 percent. There are, of course, follicular variants of both papillary and medullary carcinoma, but these behave as papillary and medullary cancer, not as the follicular type. Other, much rarer variants of follicular cancer include the type resembling renal clear cell carcinoma and the insular type of thyroid cancer, which is an aggressive form of follicular carcinoma with a solid growth pattern. Vascular invasion and hematogenous metastasis are usual with follicular cancer, so that intrathyroidal foci from lymphatic spread would not occur, although they are very common with papillary cancer. Absence of ground-glass nuclei or well-formed papillae or psammoma bodies differentiates follicular from papillary carcinoma.

295. The answer is D. *(Robbins, 4/e. pp 1217–1218, 1224–1226.)* Graves' disease, or diffuse toxic goiter, is one of the three most common disorders associated with thyrotoxicosis or hyperthyroidism (the other two are toxic multinodular goiter and toxic adenoma). This hyperfunctioning and hyperplastic diffuse goiter is accompanied by infiltrative ophthalmopathy, including exophthalmos or proptosis—only seen in Graves' disease. Dermopathy or pretibial "myxedema" is present in up to 15 percent of cases. Graves' disease is an autoimmune form of goiter caused by thyroid-stimulating immunoglobulins or thyroid-stimulating hormone receptor antibodies. Autoantibodies to TSH receptor antigens are produced because of a defect in antigen-specific suppressor T cells. The antibodies bind to TSH receptors on thyroid follicular cells and function as TSH, with resultant thyroid growth and hyperfunction. Such antibodies can be identified in almost all cases of Graves' disease. Cardiac manifestations include tachycardia, cardiomegaly, and occasional arrhythmias (atrial fibrillation), and these are often early features. Diffuse toxic goiter is associated with HLA-DR3 genotype.

296. The answer is B. *(Anderson, 9/e. pp 1546–1549.)* The histologic appearance of colloid storage goiter generally includes abnormally large, colloid-filled follicles compressing the intervening small or normal-sized follicles that contain very little colloid. The epithelium of the follicles is predominantly flat cuboidal, with occasional epithelial papillary structures protruding into the follicles. In primary hyperplasia with Graves' disease, the follicular epithelium is tall, with papillary infoldings and peripheral vacuolation of the colloid. Riedel's struma appears as a marked fibrous tissue replacement of the normal thyroid histology. In Hashimoto's thyroiditis, only remnants of thyroid follicles and epithelial cells are found in sheets of lymphocytes with germinal centers.

297. The answer is D. *(Robbins, 4/e. pp 1269–1271.)* Thymomas are tumors arising from thymic epithelial cells and form one of the most common mediastinal neoplasms, especially in the anterosuperior mediastinum. There is a scant or rich lymphocytic infiltrate of T cells, which are not neoplastic, although their size and prominent nucleoli may cause histologic confusion with lymphoma. About 90 percent of thymomas are benign and occur at a mean age of 50 years. They are very rare in children. They may be asymptomatic or cause pressure effects of dysphagia, dyspnea, or vena caval compression. Associated systemic disorders include myasthenia gravis, hematologic cytopenias, collagen vascular disease (lupus), and hypogammaglobulinemia. Malignant thymomas show infiltration and capsular invasion plus pleural implants or distant metastasis.

298. The answer is C. *(Henry, 18/e. pp 310–311. Robbins, 4/e. pp 1207–1210.)* The constellation of cartilaginous-periosteal soft tissue growth of the distal extremities (acromegaly) and growth of the skull and face bones is characteristic of hypersecretion of growth hormone (GH) from an anterior pituitary adenoma. GH modulates the production of hepatic somatomedin (sulfation factor). Somatomedins are small peptides that act on the target organs after being synthesized under the influence of growth hormone. They have insulin-like properties but are immunologically distinct from insulin. In addition to acral-skeletal expansion, patients with hyperpituitarism of the adult-onset variety (occurring after epiphyseal plate closure) have organomegaly, including increased size of the heart, kidneys, liver, and spleen. Cardiac failure is usually the mechanism of death.

299. The answer is C. *(Robbins, 4/e. pp 1220–1222.)* Hashimoto's (autoimmune) thyroiditis is one of the conditions of chronic thyroiditis. It is not that uncommon in the United States. The stroma is permeated by a dense lymphoplasmacytic infiltrate with lymphoid follicles (germinal centers) that distorts and transforms thyroid follicles into collections of acidophilic cells (oncocytes, Hürthle-like cells). Not uncommonly, patients develop hypothyroidism as a result of follicle disruption, and the manifestations consist of fatigue, myxedema, cold intolerance, hair coarsening, and constipation. Whereas subacute (DeQuervain's) thyroiditis, Riedel's thyroiditis, and psychosomatic complaints may cause common symptoms, biopsy findings of these disorders are distinctly different from those of Hashimoto's disease.

300. The answer is E. *(Anderson, 9/e. pp 1605–1606.)* Myelolipoma is not clearly neoplastic; it is a circumscribed, yellow-red, tumorlike growth of bone marrow, composed microscopically of fat, red and white cell precursors, and megakaryocytes—a tissue resembling bone marrow surrounded by adrenal cortex. Origin appears to be in the inner zona fasciculata and it measures 0.5

to 6 cm in diameter, though it is occasionally larger. Extraadrenal myeloli-pomas may occur in the intercostal spaces and retroperitoneal or pelvic con-nective tissue. Rare adrenal myelolipomas have accompanied Cushing's syn-drome and contained adrenocortical cells, but myelolipoma is usually incidental, without symptoms. It is a benign lesion, possibly representing mesenchymal rests.

301. The answer is E. *(Robbins, 4/e. pp 1259–1260.)* Edema is not a feature of primary hyperaldosteronism (Conn's syndrome), which is characterized by weakness, hypertension, polydipsia, and polyuria. The underlying physio-logic abnormalities include alkaline urine, an elevated level of serum sodium, hypokalemic alkalosis, and excessive potassium loss by the kidneys. The level of serum aldosterone is elevated; that of plasma renin is suppressed. The elevated level of serum sodium causes expansion of the intravascular volume. A single adenoma has been described as the causative factor of pri-mary hyperaldosteronism in the majority of patients, and carcinoma, multiple adenomas, and cortical hyperplasia have been cited occasionally as causes of this syndrome.

302. The answer is D. *(Robbins, 4/e. pp 1245–1247.)* Hypocalcemia resulting from any chronic cause may lead to hyperparathyroidism. The mechanism of hypocalcemia in chronic renal failure is thought to be related to phosphate retention. Sustained parathormone release results from the chronic hypocal-cemia. The parathyroid hyperplasia under these circumstances may involve one, two, three, or all four parathyroid glands in the form of chief cell hyper-plasia, frequently with scattered nests of eosinophilic, oxyphilic cells (onco-cytes). There is an accompanying replacement of the intraglandular fat by the hyperplasia. Surgical extirpation is the treatment of choice.

303. The answer is C. *(Robbins, 4/e. pp 1243–1246.)* Primary hyperparathy-roidism (HPT), as in parathyroid adenoma, leads to more extensive bone dis-ease than is found in secondary hyperparathyroidism, as in chronic renal fail-ure. Calcium levels are generally higher in the primary form of the disease than in the secondary form, in which calcium levels are low or low-normal; accordingly, the bone lesions are more severe in primary HPT, and through a process of bone resorption and fibrous replacement, cystic spaces result (os-teitis fibrosa cystica). Repeated hemorrhages may occur in these focal le-sions, with the formation of reactive granulomas (brown tumors). This is a rare event, since hypercalcemia is actively sought out and is treated early in most medical centers. The bone lesions in secondary hyperparathyroidism are of a milder degree and consist basically of a demineralization process (osteomalacia); this can be recognized as too much osteoid without appropriate mineralization. Osteoporosis involves a loss of bone, with osteoid-mineralization reduction being proportionately reduced. Osteopetrosis (Albers-Schönberg disease, or marble bone disease) is an inherited bone disease characterized by bony sclerosis and excess bone growths with loss of marrow spaces.

304. The answer is E. *(Anderson, 9/e. p 1570.)* The parathyroid glands develop from the endodermal tissue of the dorsal diverticula of the third and fourth pharyngeal pouches and usually consist of four flattened, encapsulated, oval bodies that lie against the dorsum of the thyroid gland. The superior glands, derived from the fourth pharyngeal pouches, have an anatomic position that is more constant than that of the inferior pair. The inferior parathyroids, because they develop and move caudally with the thymus, sometimes become located below the thyroid level, and the inconstant location of these parathyroids is an important factor to consider in the search for pathologic parathyroid tissue during autopsy or surgery.

305. The answer is E. *(Robbins, 4/e. p 801.)* The syndrome of inappropriate antidiuretic hormone (SIADH) is an important cause of dilutional hyponatremia that has been identified in tumors of the thymus gland, malignant lymphoma, and pancreatic neoplasms. It occurs predominantly, however, as a result of ectopic secretion of ADH by oat cell carcinomas of the lung. Since the tumor cells per se are autonomously producing ADH, there is no feedback inhibition from the hypothalamic osmoreceptors, and the persistent ADH effect on the renal tubules causes water retention even with concentrated urine. Hence the term *inappropriate ADH* arises. Laboratory findings of the syndrome include low plasma sodium levels (dilutional hyponatremia), low plasma osmolality, and high urine osmolality caused by disproportionate solute excretion without water.

306–309. The answers are: 306-A, 307-D, 308-B, 309-B. *(Robbins, 4/e. pp 1233–1240.)* Papillary carcinoma is the most common type of thyroid cancer and has the best prognosis, although lymphatic invasion is usual, which accounts for both the common metastasis to cervical lymph nodes and for the multifocal intrathyroidal spread. About 50 percent of all papillary thyroid carcinomas show follicular differentiation (follicular variants), but their biologic behavior is that of papillary carcinoma with very slow growth and long survival. Psammoma bodies are found in about 40 percent of papillary tumors (stippled calcification on x-ray), and nuclei often show characteristic clearing or ground-glass appearance. Papillary carcinoma has been related to irradiation of the head and neck in early life.

Hematogenous metastasis to brain, bone, or lungs is the usual mode of spread of follicular carcinoma, which, when well differentiated, may be confused with follicular adenoma except for invasion of blood vessels or capsule.

Medullary carcinoma of the thyroid (MCT) originates from the parafollicular C cells. It occurs in both sporadic and familial forms; the latter occurs before 30 years of age and is associated with pheochromocytomas and parathyroid hyperplasia or adenoma (Sipple's syndrome, MEN IIa). The parafollicular cells secrete calcitonin and carcinoembryonic antigen and, occasionally, ACTH, prostaglandin, serotonin, or bradykinin. Measurements of elevated serum calcitonin are useful in both diagnosis and prognosis, especially in familial settings, where family members should be screened for elevated serum levels. Follicular variants are rare but amyloid stromal deposits are frequent in MCT, which can have an indolent or aggressive course.

310–313. The answers are: 310-E, 311-D, 312-A, 313-B. *(Anderson, 9/e. pp 1526–1527, 1529, 1599–1605.)* Panhypopituitarism results from destruction of at least 75 percent of the anterior pituitary. This destruction usually is caused by tumors (e.g., metastatic carcinoma of the breast or lung) and infarction, but destruction can also be caused by inflammatory disorders, abscesses, granulomas (giant-cell granulomas of older women), and histiocytic infiltrates. *Simmonds' disease*—the eponym for the classic clinical syndrome caused by panhypopituitarism in the adult—involves insufficiency of the gonads, thyroid, and adrenals and is secondary to the absence of stimulation by the respective trophic hormones.

Sheehan's syndrome consists of symptoms of pituitary failure that occur as the result of infarction of the pituitary because of postpartum hemorrhage or other types of massive hemorrhage. In Sheehan's syndrome the pituitary infarction frequently occurs in the presence of intravascular coagulopathy of pregnancy.

Hand-Schüller-Christian disease (HSC) features histiocytic infiltrates in the pituitary and xanthomatous deposits in the skull and dura. Because the infundibular portion of the pituitary may be involved in HSC, the disease may cause diabetes insipidus in children as the pituitary is subjected to bony encasement with destruction of the nerve tracts in the neurohypophysis.

Before the age of 10, Cushing's syndrome is probably most often related to adrenal carcinoma, a tumor present in at least 50 percent of cases, while most of the remaining cases are associated with adrenocortical hyperplasia. After the age of 10, zona fasciculata hyperplasia accounts for approximately 70 percent of cases. In the adult, adrenocortical carcinoma is responsible for only 10 percent of the cases of Cushing's syndrome. Adrenal carcinomas are differentiated from adenomas by capsular or vascular invasion and metastasis.

Primary carcinoma of the anterior pituitary is not only rare but is rather undifferentiated, so that the cell type cannot be identified. However, most cases are of chromophobe origin; therefore, hormonal elaboration is very rare. It is difficult to differentiate the carcinoma from an adenoma and very local invasion is also unreliable; thus, metastasis is the only valid criterion of malignancy.

314–317. The answers are: 314-E, 315-B, 316-C, 317-D. *(Robbins, 4/e. pp 1210, 1212–1213, 1246–1247, 1259, 1263–1265.)* In secondary hyperparathyroidism, the excess secretion of parathormone (PTH) in chronic renal insufficiency is characterized by high serum phosphate and low, normal, or subnormal calcium values. Since the failing kidney is not able to synthesize 1α,25-dihydroxycholecalciferol, the most active form of vitamin D, this deficiency leads to poor absorption of calcium from the gut and relative hypocalcemia, which stimulates PTH oversecretion. Chronic renal failure is the most important cause, but secondary hyperparathyroidism also occurs in vitamin D deficiency, malabsorption syndromes, and pseudohypoparathyroidism.

Tumors of the adrenal medulla include pheochromocytoma, neuroblastoma, and ganglioneuroma. Pheochromocytoma usually occurs sporadically, but also in familial syndromes, two of which are part of MEN type II. It comprises tumors of thyroid (medullary carcinoma) and of adrenal medulla (pheochromocytoma) and chief cell hyperplasia of the parathyroids. The familial form is Sipple's syndrome (MEN type IIa) in which pheochromocytomas are bilateral in 60 to 100 percent of cases. MEN IIb includes thyroid carcinoma (medullary), pheochromocytoma, and associated neurologic abnormalities and mucosal neuromas.

Nelson's syndrome occurs following bilateral adrenalectomy for Cushing's disease; it is marked by an invasive, inoperable, hormone-secreting pituitary corticotroph adenoma. With lack of adrenal feedback control, the adenoma may release large amounts of ACTH and melanocyte-stimulating peptides into the blood, resulting in marked brown melanin pigmentation in the skin.

Hyperprolactinemia is the most common hypersecretory endocrinopathy caused by a pituitary tumor—a prolactin-producing eosinophilic adenoma. In women, an amenorrhea-galactorrhea syndrome results; in men, there may be loss of libido because of mass effect with inhibition of gonadotropin secretion or effects. Since other causes of hyperprolactinemia exist, including lesions in the hypothalamus, estrogen therapy, and drugs such as methyldopa, diagnosis of a prolactinoma requires evidence of an anterior lobe mass and elevated plasma levels of prolactin.

Genitourinary System

DIRECTIONS: Each question below contains five suggested responses. Select the **one best** response to each question.

318. The photomicrograph below depicts a biopsy of the uterine cervix that was done following an abnormal Pap smear report. This histologic section shows

(A) condyloma acuminatum
(B) carcinoma in situ
(C) dysplasia
(D) cervical intraepithelial neoplasia
(E) squamous metaplasia

319. A middle-aged man comes to you with the single presenting symptom of occasional hematuria of very recent onset. The most probable cause is

(A) acute pyelonephritis
(B) nephroblastoma
(C) renal cell carcinoma
(D) mesoblastic nephroma
(E) renal pelvic urothelial tumor

320. All the following statements are true of urinary calculi EXCEPT that

(A) they are more common in males
(B) they are bilateral in 40 percent of cases
(C) they are radiopaque in about 90 percent of cases
(D) they may be associated with *Pseudomonas* infections
(E) the incidence is increased in leukemia

321. A linear pattern of immunoglobulin deposition along the glomerular basement membrane that can be demonstrated by immunofluorescence is typical of

(A) lupus nephritis
(B) diabetic glomerulopathy
(C) Goodpasture's syndrome
(D) Goldblatt's kidney
(E) renal vein thrombosis

322. What is the correct treatment for a patient who has hypertension secondary to unilateral renal artery stenosis when the contralateral kidney shows severe arteriolonephrosclerosis?

(A) Ureteral reimplantation
(B) Removal of the kidney supplied by the stenotic artery
(C) Repair of the renal artery stenosis and ipsilateral nephrectomy
(D) Repair of the renal artery stenosis and contralateral nephrectomy
(E) Nonsurgical management

323. An adult medical laboratory technician recovering from hepatitis B develops hematuria, proteinuria, and red cell casts in the urine. Which of the following would best describe the changes occurring within the kidney in this patient?

(A) Plasma cell interstitial nephritis
(B) IgG linear fluorescence along the glomerular basement membrane
(C) Granular deposits of antibodies in the glomerular basement membrane
(D) Diffuse glomerular basement membrane thickening by subepithelial immune deposits
(E) Nodular hyaline glomerulosclerosis

324. Marked glomerular basement membrane thickening, as shown in the photomicrograph below, may be seen in all the following conditions EX-CEPT

(A) lupus nephritis
(B) membranous glomerulonephritis
(C) diabetes mellitus
(D) acute pyelonephritis
(E) renal vein thrombosis

325. The gross appearance of the kidney shown is most compatible with which of the following conditions?

(A) Cystic renal dysplasia
(B) Acute pyelonephritis
(C) Chronic pyelonephritis
(D) Acute glomerulonephritis
(E) Chronic glomerulonephritis

326. All the following characteristics are associated with the disorder depicted in the photograph below EXCEPT

(A) massive unilateral enlargement
(B) autosomal dominant inheritance in adult form
(C) autosomal recessive inheritance in childhood form
(D) hepatic cysts in childhood form
(E) possible association with berry aneurysms

327. A sexually active man who has had a negative evaluation for gonococcal infection and who complains of persistent dysuria but no other symptoms should be considered to have

(A) prostatic hypertrophy
(B) epididymitis
(C) orchitis
(D) nonspecific urethritis
(E) renal stones

328. Which of the following is sufficiently different from the others to be discriminated by histologic examination only?

(A) Bowen's disease
(B) Squamous cell carcinoma in situ
(C) Erythroplasia of Queyrat
(D) Bowenoid papulosis
(E) Human papilloma virus (HPV) condyloma

329. A 46-year-old woman undergoes an abdominal hysterectomy for
a "fibroid" uterus. The surgeon re-
quests a frozen section on the tumor, which is deferred because of
the lesion's degree of cellularity.
Which of the following criteria will
be used by the pathologist in deter-
mining benignancy versus malignancy in permanent sections?

(A) Mitotic rate
(B) Cell pleomorphism
(C) Cell necrosis
(D) Nucleocytoplasmic (NC) ratio
(E) Tumor size

330. A 23-year-old woman with an
abnormal Pap smear undergoes a
cervical biopsy. The results are read
as "CIN-2." What is the meaning of
this report?

(A) Cervical carcinoma, grade II
(B) Cervical carcinoma, stage II
(C) Cervical inflammation; repeat in
    2 months
(D) Carcinoma in situ
(E) Moderate dysplasia

331. The photomicrograph below is of a section from a testis removed from
the inguinal region of a man aged 25. Which of the following statements is
true regarding the condition illustrated?

(A) It occurs in 5 percent of the adult male population
(B) Teratoma is the most common malignancy to arise
(C) Risk of associated malignancy is reduced by orchiopexy
(D) There is increased risk of malignancy in the contralateral testis
(E) Both Leydig and Sertoli cells are reduced in number

332. The condition shown in the photomicrograph, malacoplakia of the urinary bladder, is considered to be associated with

(A) tuberculosis
(B) urothelial carcinoma
(C) schistosomiasis
(D) staphylococcal infections
(E) defects in phagocytosis

333. The ovarian lesion in the photomicrograph below is

(A) chronic salpingitis
(B) an ectopic pregnancy
(C) a granulosa cell tumor
(D) a cystic teratoma
(E) metastatic squamous cell carcinoma

334. A woman harboring endometrial adenocarcinoma nearly always has antecedent

(A) obesity
(B) diabetes mellitus
(C) endometrial polyps
(D) endometrial hyperplasia
(E) systemic hypertension

335. A 10-year-old boy has a bout of ordinary upper respiratory infection followed within 36 h by an episode of hematuria. There are no joint symptoms, gastrointestinal symptoms, petechiae, or rashes. To confirm the suspicion of Berger's disease, which of the following is indicated?

(A) Examination of urinary sediment
(B) Renal scan
(C) Renal biopsy immunofluorescence
(D) Creatinine clearance
(E) Intravenous pyelogram

336. Vaginal adenosis precedes the development of which of the following?

(A) Condyloma acuminatum
(B) Cervical carcinoma
(C) Clear cell carcinoma
(D) Carcinoma of the endometrium
(E) Squamous carcinoma of the vagina

337. The majority of malignant tumors of the ovary take their origin from

(A) surface epithelium
(B) urogenital stem cells
(C) ovarian germ cells
(D) stromal cells
(E) hilar cells

338. Ovarian cystadenomas or cystadenocarcinomas (serous or mucinous)

(A) always produce androgens
(B) seldom are bilateral
(C) can be papillary
(D) usually occur during pregnancy
(E) are extremely rare

339. Acute tubular necrosis (ATN) is a fairly common renal lesion and is associated with all the following EXCEPT

(A) red cell casts in the urine
(B) proteinuria
(C) proximal tubular damage in toxic ATN
(D) oliguria
(E) acute renal failure

340. Primary germ cell tumors of the testis occur predominantly in the younger male with the exception of

(A) embryonal carcinoma
(B) spermatocytic seminoma
(C) polyembryoma
(D) choriocarcinoma
(E) teratocarcinoma

341. In the list below, the ovarian tumor with the highest degree of bilateral involvement is

(A) endometrioid carcinoma
(B) serous cystadenoma
(C) mucinous cystadenoma
(D) mucinous cystadenocarcinoma
(E) serous cystadenocarcinoma

342. A small, palpable, well-circumscribed nodule in the epididymis is most likely to be

(A) androblastoma
(B) tuberculous granuloma
(C) carcinoma
(D) adenomatoid tumor
(E) adrenocortical rest

343. The cells in the photomicrograph below were the predominant type in a Papanicolaou stained smear of the lateral vaginal wall from a 66-year-old woman. The cell pattern shows a predominance of

(A) superficial squamous cells
(B) intermediate squamous cells
(C) parabasal squamous cells
(D) malignant squamous cells
(E) histiocytes

344. Which of the following genera is most responsible for venereal disease in women in the United States?

(A) *Calymmatobacterium*
(B) *Campylobacter*
(C) *Chlamydia*
(D) *Neisseria*
(E) *Haemophilus*

345. All the following statements are true regarding transitional cell carcinoma of the bladder EXCEPT that

(A) it is more common in men than in women
(B) it is associated with infection by *Schistosoma haematobium*
(C) it is associated with cigarette smoking
(D) it shows increased incidence in aniline dye workers
(E) it tends to recur after excision, regardless of grade

346. A patient being investigated for hematuria and proteinuria has a renal biopsy that shows changes in the glomeruli as depicted below. All the following diseases can be associated with changes seen in this biopsy EXCEPT

(A) bacterial endocarditis
(B) anaphylactoid purpura
(C) systemic lupus erythematosus
(D) hereditary nephritis (Alport's syndrome)
(E) diabetes mellitus

347. Acute poststreptococcal glomerulonephritis usually does all the following EXCEPT

(A) follow infection with group A beta-hemolytic streptococci
(B) follow a streptococcal infection in less than 5 days
(C) have a better prognosis in children than in adults
(D) show low serum complement levels (hypocomplementemia)
(E) exhibit elevation of antistreptolysin O (ASO) titer

348. Diseases of the urinary tract occurring with increased frequency in patients with diabetes mellitus include all the following EXCEPT

(A) nodular or intercapillary glomerulosclerosis
(B) nephrotic syndrome
(C) atherosclerosis of the renal artery
(D) renal papillary necrosis
(E) acute pyelonephritis

---

349. The photomicrograph below shows evidence of glomerular fibrin deposition. This histopathology is a supplemental finding in a 2-year-old child who has a history of abdominal pain and bloody diarrhea, followed by acute glomerulonephritis, Coombs'-negative severe hemolytic anemia, and renal failure. The likely diagnoses might include

(A) lupus erythematosus
(B) acute poststreptococcal glomerulonephritis
(C) lipoid nephrosis
(D) hemolytic-uremic syndrome
(E) bacterial endocarditis

350. True statements concerning the hemolytic-uremic syndrome (HUS) in young children include all the following EXCEPT

(A) endothelial injury is an initiating pathologic event
(B) prior infection with *E. coli* is common
(C) hypertension exists in about half the patients
(D) involvement of the CNS is a dominant feature
(E) acute, anuric renal failure occurs in over 50 percent of cases

351. Components of diabetic glomerulopathy include all the following EXCEPT

(A) diffuse glomerulosclerosis
(B) nodular glomerulosclerosis
(C) thickening of capillary basement membranes
(D) mesangial proliferation
(E) fibrin thrombi

352. All the following renal disorders are associated with the nephrotic syndrome EXCEPT

(A) membranous glomerulonephritis
(B) lipoid nephrosis
(C) membranoproliferative glomerulonephritis
(D) acute tubular necrosis
(E) focal segmental glomerulosclerosis

353. All the following renal diseases cause hypertension EXCEPT

(A) small, bilateral renal infarcts
(B) renal artery arteriosclerosis
(C) fibromuscular dysplasia of the renal artery
(D) hydronephrosis
(E) pyelonephritis

354. A major risk factor for squamous carcinoma of the cervix is now considered to be

(A) early sexual activity
(B) multiple sexual partners
(C) human papilloma virus types 16/18
(D) herpes simplex virus type 2
(E) *Chlamydia trachomatis*

355. A young woman with lower pelvic pain, menometrorrhagia, and a negative β-hCG test undergoes uterine dilatation and curettage. The pathology report on the endometrial samples states, "Compatible with decidualized gestational hyperplasia, no chorionic villi present." The next step would be to

(A) repeat the β-hCG test
(B) discharge the patient
(C) consider ectopic pregnancy
(D) consider appendicitis
(E) consider pelvic inflammatory disease

356. Carcinoma of the prostate tends to do all the following EXCEPT

(A) be adenocarcinoma
(B) arise in the posterior lobe
(C) cause elevation of serum acid phosphatase
(D) be estrogen-dependent
(E) form osteoblastic metastases

357. A female patient is being treated with penicillin for acute salpingitis and pelvic inflammatory disease without benefit. Which of the following organisms should now be considered in the differential diagnosis?

(A) *Treponema pallidum*
(B) *Neisseria gonorrhoeae*
(C) *Chlamydia trachomatis*
(D) Adenoviruses
(E) Herpesviruses

358. An 18-month-old infant is evaluated for generalized tissue edema and ascites. Urinalysis shows numerous hyaline casts and lipid droplets. Total plasma protein and albumin are markedly decreased, whereas total lipids are increased. A light micrograph of a renal biopsy glomerulus is shown below. Statements applicable to this disorder include that

(A) the problem is hepatic, not renal
(B) electron microscopy is diagnostic
(C) light microscopy is diagnostic
(D) exacerbations are uncommon
(E) response to steroid therapy is poor

359. Cystic hyperplasia of the endometrium is associated with all the following EXCEPT

(A) occurrence at or just before menopause
(B) increased estrogen administration or production
(C) excessive uterine bleeding
(D) secretory cells lining the cystically dilated glands
(E) functioning granulosa-theca cell tumors

360. A major role in the exclusion of albumin from the ultrafiltrate in the normal human glomerulus is played by

(A) sodium-potassium ATPase
(B) parietal epithelium
(C) endothelial fenestrations
(D) proteoglycans
(E) podocytes

361. Common outcomes of the uterine abnormality illustrated below include all the following EXCEPT

(A) malignant change
(B) cystic degeneration
(C) calcification
(D) rapid enlargement during pregnancy
(E) atrophy after menopause

362. The photomicrograph below shows an abnormal renal tubular epithelial cell in a urinary specimen from a very ill renal transplant patient. The disease diagnosed is associated with all the following EXCEPT

(A) interstitial pneumonitis
(B) hepatitis
(C) a herpesvirus
(D) gastrointestinal ulcers
(E) detection of antigen in 1 to 3 weeks

363. A significant role in vascular permeability, particularly in the renal glomerulus, is played by

(A) collagen type IV
(B) desmin
(C) fibronectin
(D) podocytes
(E) polyanions

364. The photomicrograph below shows a section through a testis removed from a 30-year-old man with acute scrotal pain. True statements regarding this condition include that

(A) infection is usually by the hematogenous route
(B) sterility is a rare complication
(C) the epididymis is usually spared
(D) *Chlamydia trachomatis* is a common pathogen
(E) interstitial cells of Leydig are destroyed

365. In vaginal fluid the most conclusive evidence of coitus is

(A) alkaline phosphatase
(B) acid phosphatase
(C) prostatic acid phosphatase
(D) p30 antigen
(E) prostatic specific antigen

366. The kidney shown in the photomicrograph below exhibits a tumor that has originated in the upper pole. Correct statements about this tumor include all the following EXCEPT that

(A) it is sometimes associated with polycythemia
(B) it is sometimes associated with tuberous sclerosis
(C) it may produce glucocorticoids
(D) it originates from proximal convoluted tubular cells
(E) it occurs predominantly in the sixth decade

367. Primary malignant neoplasms of the vagina include all the following EXCEPT

(A) sarcoma botryoides
(B) clear cell carcinoma
(C) squamous carcinoma
(D) vaginal adenosis
(E) rhabdomyosarcoma

DIRECTIONS: Each group of questions below consists of lettered headings followed by a set of numbered items. For each numbered item select the **one** lettered heading with which it is **most** closely associated. Each lettered heading may be used **once, more than once, or not at all.**

Questions 368–371

Match the renal disorders with the pathologic findings with which they are most likely to be associated.

(A) Hyalinized glomeruli
(B) Splitting of the glomerular basement membranes
(C) Diffuse thickening of capillary walls
(D) Mesangial deposits and subepithelial "humps"
(E) Glomerular epithelial crescents

368. Membranoproliferative glomerulonephritis

369. Membranous glomerulonephritis

370. Poststreptococcal glomerulonephritis (PSGN)

371. Goodpasture's syndrome

DIRECTIONS: The groups of questions below consist of four lettered headings followed by a set of numbered items. For each numbered item select

A	if the item is associated with	(A) **only**
B	if the item is associated with	(B) **only**
C	if the item is associated with	**both** (A) and (B)
D	if the item is associated with	**neither** (A) nor (B)

Each lettered heading may be used **once, more than once, or not at all.**

Questions 372–376

(A) Choriocarcinoma
(B) Hydatidiform mole
(C) Both
(D) Neither

372. Production of alpha-fetoprotein

373. Malignancy of trophoblastic cells

374. Occurrence in 1 in 2000 pregnancies in U.S.

375. Primary germ cell tumor of testis

376. Considerable elevation in titers of human chorionic gonadotropin (hCG)

Questions 377–380

(A) Minimal change disease (lipoid nephrosis)
(B) Focal segmental glomerulosclerosis
(C) Both
(D) Neither

377. Association with nephrotic syndrome

378. Association with AIDS

379. Very good response to steroid therapy

380. Deposition of IgM and C3

Questions 381–384

Match the listed clinical or pathologic characteristics with the appropriate ovarian tumor.

(A) Benign ovarian fibroma
(B) Endometrioid tumor
(C) Brenner tumor
(D) Granulosa-theca cell tumor
(E) Metastatic signet-ring cancer

381. Approximately 20 percent of all ovarian cancers

382. Endometrial hyperplasia

383. Ascites and pleural effusion

384. Gastrointestinal carcinoma

Questions 385–388

Match each disease with the pathologic finding that is most characteristic.

(A) Malignant nephrosclerosis
(B) Benign nephrosclerosis
(C) Preeclampsia
(D) Analgesic abuse nephropathy
(E) Systemic lupus erythematosus

385. Hyaline arteriolosclerosis

386. Swollen glomerular endothelial cells

387. Papillary necrosis

388. Arteriolar fibrinoid necrosis

Genitourinary System
Answers

318. The answer is A. *(Richart, Cancer 60:1951–1959, 1987. Robbins, 4/e. pp 1135, 1142–1143.)* Cervical condylomata, particularly flat condylomata, although benign are considered to be precursors of cervical intraepithelial neoplasia (CIN), which comprises both dysplasia and carcinoma in situ (CIS). Histologically, these condylomata consist of connective tissue stroma covered by hyperplastic epithelium with prominent perinuclear cytoplasmic vacuolization (koilocytosis). Koilocytotic cells are characteristic of human papilloma virus (HPV) infection. More than 50 genotypes of HPV are known at present, and condylomata acuminata are associated with types 6/11 while HPV types 16/18 are usually present in CIN. Following an abnormal Pap smear report suggesting condyloma, CIN, or possible invasive carcinoma, workup of the patient should include colposcopy, multiple cervical punch biopsies, and endocervical curettage to distinguish patients who have invasive cancer, CIN, or flat condylomata.

319. The answer is E. *(Robbins, 4/e. p 1078.)* A middle-aged patient is highly unlikely to have either of the predominantly childhood tumors nephroblastoma (Wilms' tumor) or mesoblastic nephroma (benign hamartoma). Mesoblastic nephroma, which may be seen in the first year of life, has caused difficulty in differential diagnosis from Wilms' tumor in children. Acute pyelonephritis features signs of acute infection with flank pain, pyuria, fever, and a high bacterial colony count in urine. Renal cell carcinoma is unlikely to cause hematuria until far advanced with invasion of the collecting system. Urothelial renal pelvic tumors cause hematuria early, even when quite small. They form 5 to 10 percent of primary renal tumors and range from apparently benign papillomas to papillary or anaplastic carcinomas. There may be multicentric involvement of ureters or bladder. Diagnosis is by x-ray and cytologic examination of at least three voided urine specimens; malignant cells are not found if the ureter is obstructed by tumor, or if the cells are degenerate or mildly atypical, as in papilloma. Prognosis is not very good for high-grade infiltrating tumors and is very poor for the squamous cell variant (about 15 percent of pelvic tumors); therefore, early diagnosis is paramount.

320. The answer is B. *(Robbins, 4/e. pp 1073–1074.)* Urinary calculi are a common problem and may arise at any level of the urinary tract, but mainly in the kidney. They are more common in males and most patients are over 30 years of age. Urinary calculi are unilateral in 80 percent of cases, and 90 percent are radiopaque since most contain calcium oxalate or calcium phosphate. Other constituents include magnesium ammonium phosphate, cystine, and uric acid. Urate stones are radiolucent and are increased in hyperuricemia due to gout and in conditions with rapid cell turnover such as leukemia. Urea-splitting organisms such as *Pseudomonas* predispose to calculi.

321. The answer is C. *(Robbins, 4/e. pp 1031–1032.)* In Goodpasture's syndrome, circulating antibodies reactive with the glomerular basement membrane will bind in a linear pattern along the entire length of the glomerular basement membrane, which is their specific antigen. IgG is deposited in the basement membrane, along with complement. There are focal interruptions of the glomerular basement membrane as well, along with deposits of fibrin, as seen with electron microscopy.

322. The answer is D. *(Robbins, 4/e. pp 1068–1069.)* In a patient with a surgically correctable lesion of the renal artery, the corresponding kidney, which is potentially the less damaged one, should be saved. The contralateral kidney may be severely affected with arteriolonephrosclerosis and could perpetuate the hypertension if not removed. In a patient with parenchymal renal disease leading to hypertension, such as pyelonephritis, removal of the affected kidney may relieve the hypertension.

323. The answer is C. *(Robbins, 4/e. pp 1024–1036.)* Glomerular injury caused by circulating antigen-antibody complexes is a secondary effect from a nonprimary renal source. Numerous clinical examples exist of a serum sickness–like nephritis as a consequence of systemic infection, with classic clinical models such as syphilis, hepatitis B, malaria, and bacterial endocarditis leading to renal disease. Immune complexes to antigens from any of these sources are circulating within the vascular system and become entrapped within the filtration system of the glomerular basement membranes. This can be seen as granular bumpy deposits by immunofluorescence within the basement membranes of the glomeruli. Linear fluorescence, on the other hand, is seen in primary antiglomerular basement membrane disease, wherein antibodies are directed against the glomerular basement membrane itself. Plasma cell interstitial nephritis is seen in immunologic rejection of transplanted kidneys. Nodular glomerulosclerosis is an effect of diabetes mellitus. The presence of red blood cell casts in the urine nearly always indicates that there has been glomerular injury but is not specific for any given cause. Glomerular basement membrane thickening caused by subepithelial immune deposits is seen in membranous glomerulonephritis. While the morphology of membranous glomerulonephritis is different from that of nephritis caused by circulating antigen-antibody complexes (immune complexes), there are similarities in the pathogenesis in that both disorders may be a consequence of or in association with infections such as hepatitis B, syphilis, and malaria. Other causes for membranous glomerulonephritis include reactions to penicillamine, gold, and certain malignancies such as malignant melanoma.

324. The answer is D. (*Robbins, 4/e. pp 198–200, 1043.*) The thickening of the basement membrane in systemic lupus erythematosus and membranous glomerulonephritis is thought to result from deposition of immune complexes. The pathogenesis of this same lesion in diabetes mellitus and renal vein thrombosis is unknown. Electron-dense deposits are classically seen in a subendothelial position on the glomerular basement membrane but may be subepithelial as well in some cases.

325. The answer is C. (*Robbins, 4/e. pp 1019, 1042–1043, 1055–1057.*) The kidney shown is typical of chronic pyelonephritis with dilatation of the renal pelvis, clubbing of the calyces, and irregular reduction in parenchymal mass. Chronic pyelonephritis is an asymmetric, irregularly scarring process that may be unilateral or bilateral. Microscopically, there is atrophy and dilatation of tubules with colloid in some tubules. Chronic inflammation and fibrosis occur in the cortex and medulla. Chronic glomerulonephritis causes bilateral, symmetrically shrunken and scarred kidneys. Histologic changes depend on the stage of the disease. Cystic dysplasia is characterized by undifferentiated mesenchyme and immature cartilage and collecting ductules.

326. The answer is A. (*Robbins, 4/e. pp 1018–1021.*) Polycystic kidney disease is a serious renal disorder that is inherited in two forms. The adult form is autosomal dominant with high penetrance of nearly 100 percent involvement of progeny who live to be older. The childhood polycystic form is autosomal recessive in inheritance. In the adult form one-third of the patients have cysts within the liver, while nearly all the childhood cases have hepatic cysts. Congenital hepatic fibrosis is associated with childhood polycystic kidney disease. In the adult form bilateral renal involvement is nearly invariable. One-third of patients with the adult form of polycystic kidney disease succumb to renal failure, while death occurs in another third as a consequence of hypertension.

327. The answer is D. (*Robbins, 4/e. pp 1095–1096.*) Nonspecific urethritis may actually be the most common cause of dysuria in sexually active males, although gonorrhea should always be excluded by laboratory examination. Causes of nonspecific urethritis include some bacteria, such as *Escherichia coli* and streptococci, but recent evidence implicates chlamydiae of the TRIC group as being perhaps the most common offending agents. The organism may take up residence in the prostate, producing chronic and active prostatitis. Prostatic hypertrophy, epididymitis, orchitis, and renal stones may cause urinary symptoms but also produce other signs and symptoms that distinguish them from nonspecific urethritis.

328. The answer is E. *(Robbins, 4/e. pp 1100–1102.)* Of all the choices given, human papilloma virus (HPV) condyloma without dysplasia is the only lesion that can be histologically discriminated from the others. The typical HPV condyloma has hyperplastic squamous mucosa that shows progressive maturation from the stratum germinativum to the surface that is often parakeratotic, without cells of dysplasia or malignancy. There often are vacuolated squamous cells in several layers of the mucosa. However, condylomas, whether arising in the female or the male genital areas, may have atypia or dysplasia or even be associated histologically with carcinoma. If present, these features must be commented upon in a pathology report. Condyloma not otherwise specified indicates that none of these disorders of growth are present along with it. Bowen's disease and erythroplasia of Queyrat are different clinical forms of squamous cell carcinoma in situ. Erythroplasia of Queyrat is a specialized form of squamous carcinoma in situ or severe dysplasia occurring on the glans penis mainly. It is characterized by a moist, macular, spreading red surface. It usually occurs in males of advanced age. Bowen's disease is also squamous carcinoma in situ but may have an association with malignancies of the viscera. Bowenoid papulosis refers to multiple, small, banal-appearing clinical papules on the vulvar or penile surfaces; it histologically shows features of Bowen's disease, and for all practical purposes cannot be distinguished from that disease on histologic grounds only. It is a rather new entity, histologically similar to carcinoma in situ, and it behaves as a self-healing and reversible lesion. Bowenoid papulosis usually occurs in young patients and is often associated with condylomas.

329. The answer is A. *(Anderson, 9/e. pp 1860–1864.)* "Fibroids" of the uterus are among the most common abnormalities seen in uteri surgically removed in the United States in women of reproductive age. They arise in the myometrium, submucosally, subserosally, and midwall, both singly and several at a time. Sharply circumscribed, they are benign, smooth muscle tumors that are firm, gray-white, and whorled on cut section. Their malignant counterpart, leiomyosarcoma of the uterus, is quite rare in the de novo state and arises even more rarely from an antecedent leiomyoma. Whereas cell pleomorphism, tissue necrosis, and cytologic atypia per se are established criteria in assessing malignancy in tumors generally, they are important to the pathologist in uterine fibroids only if mitoses are also present. Regardless of cellularity or atypicality, if 10 or more mitoses are present in 10 separate high-power microscopic fields, the lesion is leiomyosarcoma. If 5 or fewer mitoses are present in 10 fields with bland morphology, the leiomyoma is going to behave in a benign fashion. Problems arise when the mitotic counts range between 3 and 7 per 10 fields with varying degrees of cell and tissue atypicality. These equivocal lesions should be regarded by both pathologist and clinician as "gray-area" smooth muscle tumors of unpredictable biologic behavior. Fortunately, the "gray-area" leiomyoma of the uterus is rarely seen. Thus mitoses are the most important criteria in assessing malignancy in smooth muscle tumors of the uterus.

330. The answer is E. *(Robbins, 4/e. pp 1142–1144.)* Although the cervical intraepithelial neoplasia (CIN) system is not accepted by all workers in gynecology, many large centers are now using it for reporting cervical dysplasias. The system was created to circumvent and alleviate interpretation difficulties for pathologists because cervical dysplasia includes a spectrum of diseases that, in many cases, eventuate in carcinoma in situ followed by a stage of microinvasion. The squamous mucosa is examined for atypical squamous cells and the thickness of the total mucosa occupied by them. CIN-1 represents less than one-third thickness (mild dysplasia); CIN-2 represents one-third to two-thirds thickness (moderate dysplasia); CIN-3 represents two-thirds to the entire thickness occupied by abnormal cells (severe dysplasia, carcinoma in situ). It should be remembered that not all forms of cervical dysplasia inevitably go on to the next higher stage of disease—some are reversible.

331. The answer is D. *(Robbins, 4/e. pp 1103–1104, 1108–1109.)* The condition illustrated is cryptorchidism, failure of the testis to descend into the scrotum. It is present in up to 1 percent of males after puberty. The testis is small, brown, and atrophic grossly. Microscopically, the tubules are atrophic with thickened basement membranes. The interstitial cells are usually prominent and occasional focal proliferations of Sertoli cells may be seen. The incidence of malignancy is increased by a factor of 30 to 50 and this risk is greater for abdominal than for inguinal location. Seminoma is the most common malignancy. The risk of malignancy is not reduced by orchiopexy. There is a smaller but definite risk of malignancy in the contralateral, correctly placed testis.

332. The answer is E. *(Anderson, 9/e. pp 856–857. Robbins, 4/e. pp 1089–1090.)* Malacoplakia is an uncommon chronic inflammatory disease of unknown cause, characterized by soft yellow mucosal plaques, infiltration of large histiocytes containing phagolysosomes, and intracytoplasmic and extracellular laminated calcospherules, Michaelis-Gutmann (MG) bodies. While malacoplakia usually involves the mucosa of the urinary bladder, it occurs also in extravesical sites such as the colon, lungs, kidneys, prostate, and brain. It occurs with greater frequency in the immunosuppressed. Histologically, the plaques contain numerous, large, foamy or granular macrophages that are PAS-positive and often include bacterial debris. Laminated, mineralized MG bodies are also numerous in and between macrophages. The cause of malacoplakia is not clear, but it has been associated with *E. coli* infections and is thought to be due to defective removal by macrophages of phagocytosed bacteria with overloaded phagosomes and MG bodies resulting from calcium deposition on the phagosomes. In recent reports, however, cerebral malacoplakia was not associated with bacterial infection.

333. The answer is D. *(Anderson, 9/e. pp 1688–1690.)* Benign cystic teratomas constitute about 10 percent of cystic ovarian tumors. The cysts contain greasy sebaceous material mixed with a variable amount of hair. The cysts' walls contain skin and skin appendages, including sebaceous glands and hair follicles. A variety of other tissues—such as cartilage, bone, tooth, thyroid, respiratory tract epithelium, and intestinal tissue—may be found. The presence of skin and skin appendages gives the tumor its other name, "dermoid cyst." Dermoid cysts are benign, but in less than 2 percent, one element may become malignant, most frequently the squamous epithelium.

334. The answer is D. *(Robbins, 4/e. pp 1153–1155.)* Endometrial adenocarcinoma appears to be increasing in frequency in the United States, especially in younger women. It is now accepted that a high estrogen-to-progestin ratio predisposes to the development of this tumor. At menopause, estrogen in the form of estrone continues to be produced in the adrenal glands, and the amounts are directly proportional to body fat. This continues in a milieu in which progesterone is at a minimum because of noncycling. These factors explain why obese women are at an increased risk during and after menopause. Diabetes and hypertension also are associated factors, but they are more likely to be effects of obesity than isolated risk factors for developing cancer. Endometrial adenocarcinoma is nearly always preceded by endometrial hyperplasia in some form. This, of course, is not documented in every case because not every patient has had a diagnostic dilatation and curettage of the endometrium prior to development of the carcinoma. Furthermore, endometrial hyperplasia does not always lead to adenocarcinoma.

335. The answer is C. *(Robbins, 4/e. pp 1040–1041.)* Many diseases involve hematuria, and a few diseases occur in the setting of an upper respiratory infection or of upper respiratory signs and symptoms (streptococcal glomerulonephritis, Henoch-Schönlein purpura, Wegener's granulomatosis, and bacterial endocarditis with embolism), but when the hematuria follows within 1 to 1½ days of onset of an upper respiratory infection without skin lesions in a young patient, IgA nephropathy (Berger's disease) should be considered. This disease involves the deposition of IgA in the mesangium of the glomeruli. Light microscopic examination may suggest the disease, but renal biopsy immunofluorescence must be performed to confirm it. This disorder is not at all uncommon and may become recurrent, with proteinuria that may approach nephrotic syndrome proportions. Serum levels of IgA may be elevated. A small percentage of patients may progress to renal failure over a period of years.

336. The answer is C. *(Robbins, 4/e. p 1138.)* Adenocarcinomas of the vagina and cervix have existed for years but increased in young women whose mothers received diethylstilbestrol (DES) while they were pregnant. DES was used in the past to terminate an attack of threatened abortion and thereby stabilize the pregnancy. However, a side effect of this therapy proved to be a particular form of adenocarcinoma called clear cell carcinoma. This phenomenon was elucidated by Herpses and Scully in 1970. This unique adenocarcinoma was discovered in daughters between the ages of 15 and 20 of those women who had received DES. The tumor, which carries a poor prognosis, has at least three histologic patterns. One is a tubulopapillary configuration, followed by sheets of clear cells and glands lined by clear cells, and solid areas of relatively undifferentiated cells. Many of the cells have cytoplasm that protrudes into the lumen and produces a "hobnail" (nodular) appearance. Prior to the development of adenocarcinoma, a form of adenosis consisting of glands with clear cytoplasm that resembles that of the endocervix can be seen. This has been termed *vaginal adenosis* and may be a precursor of clear cell carcinoma. Clinically adenosis of the vagina is manifested by red, moist granules superimposed on the pink-white vaginal mucosa.

337. The answer is A. *(Robbins, 4/e. pp 1158–1164.)* Malignant tumors of the ovary most commonly occur between the ages of 40 and 64. These, in the main, arise from the surface epithelium, which takes its origin from cells of the müllerian system. These cells are also referred to as *surface,* or *coelomic, epithelium.* The müllerian system has the ability to form lining cells of the fallopian tubes, endometrium, and endocervical gland epithelium. Hence, many malignant tumors that take their origin from the surface coelomic epithelium of the ovary resemble these structures. Examples include the borderline serous tumor, serous cystadenocarcinoma, serous cystadenofibrocarcinoma, borderline mucinous tumor, mucinous cystadenocarcinoma, endometrioid carcinoma, undifferentiated carcinoma, malignant Brenner tumor, and clear cell adenocarcinoma. Stem cells from the urogenital ridge can give rise to any genitourinary structure. Hilar cells represent small clusters and cords of androgen-producing cells. These presumably give rise to sex cord and Sertoli-Leydig cell tumors. Stromal cell tumors include granulosa cell tumors, theca cell tumors, thecomas, and fibromas. Germ cell tumors give rise to malignant and benign teratomas, including the cystic form (dermoid cyst), dysgerminoma, endodermal sinus tumor, choriocarcinoma, and mixed germ cell tumors.

338. The answer is C. *(Robbins, 4/e. pp 1158–1163.)* Ovarian cystadenomas are common neoplasms that are bilateral in 15 to 40 percent of patients and are frequently papillary. The less malignant lesions tend to be more papillary. Ovarian cystadenomas originate in surface epithelial cells from the müllerian system. The papillae may show complex arborization with an increase in cell layers without stromal invasion; in such cases, the tumors are classified as borderline malignant because of their less aggressive clinical course. Unlike true cystadenocarcinomas, the presence of peritoneal dissemination in cystadenomas of borderline malignancy does not appear to influence the clinical course.

339. The answer is A. *(Robbins, 4/e. pp 1048–1051.)* In ATN, renal tubular damage follows toxic or ischemic injury and is the commonest cause of acute renal failure (ARF). Red blood cells and proteinaceous casts are usually present, but red cell casts are not associated and would suggest nephritis. Toxic ATN is caused by drugs, toxins, heavy metals (Hg), and organic solvents, and the tubular injury is predominant in proximal convoluted tubules, probably because this is the major site of nephrotoxin reabsorption. Ischemic ATN occurs after shock caused by severe infections, burns, or crush injuries with peripheral circulatory collapse. In ischemic ATN there is multiple focal tubular necrosis along the nephron often with rupture of basement membranes. Although urinary output in ATN often decreases to less than 400 mL per day (oliguria), up to 50 percent of patients with ATN may not have oliguria but may have increased urinary volumes.

340. The answer is B. *(Anderson, 9/e. pp 882–886.)* Most malignant germ cell tumors of the gonads, specifically the testis, typically occur in the younger man between the ages of 22 and 35. The seminoma has several types, most of which are found also within the younger ages. The classic seminoma is populated by differentiated seminiferous tubule–type epithelium with intervening lymphocytes, while the anaplastic seminoma contains an increase in mitoses and a moderate degree of anaplasia. The spermatocytic seminoma, however, occurs in older patients, often between ages 55 and 65, and is a soft, yellowish, sometimes mucoid tumor that microscopically has several cell types: classic intermediate-sized germ cells; smaller, secondary spermato-cytic-type cells; and large mononuclear and multinuclear giant cells. Polyem-bryoma and embryonal carcinoma are related, occur in the younger patient, and are less common than the seminomas. The most malignant germ cell tumor of the testis is the choriocarcinoma, which is characterized by large cy-totrophoblastic and syncytiotrophoblastic cells. Teratocarcinomas are tumors of more than one histologic type that may contain seminomatous or em-bryonal components, or both.

341. The answer is E. (*Robbins, 4/e. pp 1160–1163.*) Primary ovarian tumors have a rather high degree of bilateral involvement compared with tumors of other bilateral organs. Bilaterality could reflect either concurrent simultane-ous primary tumors or vascular and lymphatic spread from one side to the other. The ovarian tumor with the highest rate of bilaterality (70 percent) is the serous cystadenocarcinoma. Serous cystadenomas have a 30 percent rate of bilaterality, while mucinous cystadenomas are bilateral in about 5 percent of cases. In contrast, mucinous cystadenocarcinomas are bilateral in 20 per-cent of cases, and endometrioid carcinoma is higher at about 45 percent. There is a higher probability of extension of endometrioid carcinoma outside the ovaries when it presents with bilaterality.

342. The answer is D. (*Anderson, 9/e. p 891.*) The adenomatoid tumor is be-nign and is the most common tumor of the epididymis. Its origin is probably the mesothelium. It presents as a small, firm, gray-white nodule less than 5 cm in diameter; similar tumors occur in the fallopian tube, ovary, and poste-rior uterus. Histology reveals glandlike, mesothelium-lined, spaced and fi-brous connective tissue stroma with smooth muscle fibers. Androblastoma, or Sertoli cell tumor, is a sex cord testicular tumor, often benign; tuberculous epididymitis presents multiple confluent tubercles with caseation. Carcino-mas of epididymis and adjacent structures occur but are very rare. Adreno-cortical rests are common but usually too small for clinical detection.

343. The answer is C. (*Koss, 3/e. pp 182–190.*) Predominance of parabasal squamous cells in a lateral vaginal wall smear indicates low estrogen effect and atrophic epithelium, as in atrophic postmenopausal mucosa. A similar picture is seen with the relatively atrophic mucosa of prepuberty, lactation, or primary amenorrhea. Specimens for hormone evaluation should be ob-tained from the lateral vaginal wall and hormone assessment should not be made without knowing the patient's age, menstrual history, and whether she received exogenous hormones. Predominance of flat, superficial squamous cells with pyknotic nuclei indicates unopposed estrogen effect (ovulation or midcycle). Predominance of intermediate squamous cells is seen most often in the late luteal or secretory phase and in pregnancy.

344. The answer is C. *(Anderson, 9/e. pp 300, 324, 1645. Tam, N Engl J Med 310:1146, 1984.)* At least 50 percent of the infections of the uterine cervix in women in the United States today are caused by *Chlamydia trachomatis,* which is an intracellular obligate bacterium that can be identified by direct immunofluorescence using monoclonal antibodies. In addition to venereal transmission, *Chlamydia* also may cause psittacosis, trachoma, and neonatal infections. *Campylobacter* causes intestinal infections with diarrheal syndromes, while *Calymmatobacterium* causes granuloma inguinale, a venereally transmitted disease consisting of painful ulcers, which histologically shows granulomas with coccobacillary microorganisms within macrophages. The organism is antigenically related to *Klebsiella.* The gonococcus of the *Neisseria* genus causes gonorrhea but is less common than *Chlamydia.*

345. The answer is B. *(Robbins, 4/e. pp 1090–1094.)* Approximately 90 percent of carcinomas of the bladder are of transitional cell type. They are more common in men. Known etiologic factors include cigarette smoking, persistent mucosal inflammation, exposure to certain chemicals (notably beta-naphthylamine), and administration of the immunosuppressive agent cyclophosphamide (Cytoxan). Infection by *Schistosoma haematobium* is associated with squamous cell cancer. All transitional cell cancers, regardless of grade, tend to recur; the frequency of recurrence increases with the tumor grade.

346. The answer is E. *(Anderson, 9/e. p 815.)* The photomicrograph shows focal glomerulonephritis with crescent formation and focal hypercellularity involving only one portion of the glomerulus. Focal glomerulonephritis involves some glomeruli, but not all, and may involve the entire glomerulus (global) or only parts of the glomerulus (segmental). The photomicrograph demonstrates focal segmental glomerulonephritis, which may be seen in systemic diseases as well as disorders affecting only the kidney. Hypercellularity involved several mesangia with proliferation of epithelial cells lining Bowman's capsule near the damaged capillary loops. This process is referred to as *crescent formation.* The disease may be seen in bacterial endocarditis and other systemic infections. Immunologic disorders causing focal segmental glomerulonephritis may include IgA focal glomerulonephritis, systemic lupus erythematosus, polyarteritis nodosa, and Schönlein-Henoch purpura (anaphylactoid purpura). IgA focal glomerulonephritis, also known as Berger's disease, has deposits of IgA and some IgG in the involved mesangium as demonstrated by immunofluorescence. Alport's syndrome is a hereditary form of chronic renal disease that may be associated with neural deafness and death at an early age, usually less than 30. Large collections of foam cells are also seen in the renal cortex in these patients. Electron microscopy shows splitting of the glomerular basements accompanied by small, electron-dense granules.

347. The answer is B. *(Robbins, 4/e. pp 1029–1031. Rose, 2/e. pp 223–229.)* The acute nephritic syndrome (hematuria, red cell casts, proteinuria, and edema) may follow either pharyngitis or pyoderma (impetigo) in children or, less often, in adults. The latent period from onset of infection to evidence of renal disease averages 10 days with pharyngitis and 21 days with pyoderma; latency of less than 5 days suggests IgA nephropathy, benign hematuria, or exacerbation by infection of a chronic glomerulonephritis (GN). Clinically, 95 percent of children recover, but only about 60 percent of adults with the sporadic form recover promptly; some develop rapidly progressive GN and some of these develop chronic GN.

348. The answer is E. *(Robbins, 4/e. pp 1044–1047.)* Diabetes is a major cause of renal disease. It affects the glomeruli with resultant glomerulosclerosis, fibrin caps, and capsular drops. It also affects the renal vasculature, where it causes atheroma of the major renal arteries and hyaline arteriolosclerosis of both afferent and efferent arterioles. Acute infection of the renal pyramids occurs and in combination with impaired circulation to the papillae may lead to papillary necrosis. The finding at autopsy of acute pyelonephritis is increased in the diabetic, but this is thought to be due to the terminal event, and it is not firmly established that acute pyelonephritis is increased in the living diabetic population.

349. The answer is D. *(Robbins, 4/e. pp 1069, 1070.)* The group of renal diseases associated with microangiopathic hemolytic anemia includes both childhood and adult hemolytic-uremic syndrome (HUS), thrombotic thrombocytopenic purpura, and scleroderma. Endothelial injury and intravascular coagulation occur in all. HUS is characterized by acute renal failure, microangiopathic hemolytic anemia, and thrombocytopenia and is one of the main causes of acute renal failure in children. Prodromal features in children include a gastrointestinal or respiratory tract infection. Lupus erythematosus does not occur in very young children. Acute poststreptococcal glomerulonephritis occurs in older children, is a proliferative lesion, and is not usually associated with hemolytic anemia or fibrin deposition. Lipoid nephrosis shows no glomerular changes with light microscopy.

350. The answer is D. *(Anderson, 9/e. pp 826, 827. Robbins, 4/e. pp 1069, 1070.)* Endothelial injury is considered to be an initiating pathologic event, especially in HUS associated with gram-negative infections, predominantly infection with verocytotoxin-producing *E. coli.* The verocytotoxins of *E. coli,* which infects up to 75 percent of the patients, are cytotoxic to endothelium. Hypertension exists in about 50 percent of the patients, but the relative lack of CNS involvement helps to distinguish HUS from thrombotic thombocytopenic purpura in which there is usually more general involvement with thrombi formed in several organs.

351. The answer is E. *(Robbins, 4/e. pp 1044–1047.)* Thickening of the capillary basement membrane is a universal finding in diabetic kidney disease and consists of diffuse thickening as is seen in vasculopathy in other organ sites in diabetes. This has to be verified by ultrastructural examination by electron microscopy. Additionally, the mesangium widens and tubular basement membranes also thicken in diabetes. Thickening is produced by hyaline-like material, which reacts with the PAS stain. This may result from glycosylation of the proteins of the basement membrane. Thickening is probably also contributed by an increase in collagen type 4, as well as in the basement membrane glycoprotein laminen; however, the polyanionic proteoglycans are decreased. This may contribute to the increased permeability and consequent leakage of cationic proteins into the urine. Diffuse glomerulosclerosis results from an increase in the mesangial matrix as well as an increase in mesangial cells. This increase in matrix will also react with the PAS stain. Eventually, with continuing disease the glomerular tufts will become obliterated and yield a sclerosed, acidophilic tuft. At this stage the afferent and probably efferent arterioles will also be thickened and appear hyalinized.

Nodular glomerulosclerosis (Kimmelstiel-Wilson disease, intercapillary glomerulosclerosis) appears as laminated hyaline nodules at the peripheries of the glomerulus covered by what appears to be patent capillary loops. They may resemble amyloid and if they are present, amyloid stain should be done. Not always present, but highly characteristic of diabetic glomerulopathy are fibrin caps and capsular drops. The fibrin cap is a deposit that overlies a peripheral capillary within the glomerulus and consists of acidophilic deposits between the basement membrane and the endothelial cells. Capsular drops are PAS-positive proteinaceous foci that compose a thickening of the parietal layer of Bowman's capsule, giving the appearance of being free within the urinary ultrafiltrate.

352. The answer is D. *(Robbins, 4/e. pp 1033–1041.)* While many varieties of glomerulonephritis can produce the nephrotic syndrome, a few disorders will virtually always produce it. Included in the latter group are focal (segmental) glomerulosclerosis, membranous glomerulonephritis (GN), lipid nephrosis, membranoproliferative glomerulonephritis, systemic diseases (such as amyloidosis and systemic lupus erythematosus), some tumors, hepatitis B, syphilis, drugs such as penicillamine, and certain allergies. Light microscopy shows very little change in glomeruli in lipoid nephrosis, and a diffuse absence of glomerular epithelial foot processes is noted with electron microscopy. Membranoproliferative GN is characterized by an increase in mesangial cellularity accompanied by splitting of the glomerular basement membranes ("double contour"). Membranous GN shows electron-dense deposits of immunoglobulin in the subepithelial portion of the basement membrane. The nephrotic syndrome includes massive albuminuria with significant loss of protein (more than 3 to 5 g of protein) in 24 h, consequent reduced plasma albumin (less than 3 g/dL), hyperlipidemia, and anasarca (generalized edema).

353. The answer is A. *(Robbins, 4/e. pp 1062–1071.)* Many pathologic processes affecting the kidney can lead to hypertension. The three main categories are renovascular, renal parenchymal, and urinary tract obstruction. The renin-angiotensin system has been implicated in renovascular hypertension but has not been proved to be of etiologic importance in the other two categories. The most common parenchymal diseases leading to hypertension are pyelonephritis and hydronephrosis. Large infarcts of one kidney can cause hypertension.

354. The answer is C. *(Richart, Cancer 60:1951–1959, 1987. Robbins, 4/e. p 1142.)* Cervical squamous cell cancer and its precursors (dysplasia) are considered to be sexually transmitted diseases. Women having sexual intercourse at an early age or with multiple male partners, particularly those with penile condylomas, are at high risk for development of genital tract squamous neoplasms. Herpes simplex virus (HSV) type 2 was considered an important cause, but is now thought to have a role only in conjunction with human papilloma virus (HPV) types 16/18. Existence of the genome of HPV types 6, 11, 16, 18, 31, and 33 has been documented by DNA hybridization methods in several genital lesions including condylomas, cervical intraepithelial neoplasia (CIN) carcinoma in situ, and invasive cervical cancer. In most studies HPV 6 and 11 were confined to lesions with a good prognosis such as condylomas and mild dysplasia (CIN I), whereas HPV 16 and 18 were found predominantly in CIN III (severe dysplasia and carcinoma in situ) and in invasive carcinoma.

355. The answer is A. *(Robbins, 4/e. pp 1171–1172.)* Ectopic pregnancy is a potentially life-threatening condition if it is not treated by removal before rupture and hemorrhage with fatal exsanguination. The most common location for extrauterine implantation is the fallopian tube (more than 85 percent of cases), with rare implantation in the ovary or abdomen. If the tubal implantation has existed from 1 to 4 weeks, the β-hCG test result is likely to be negative; thus a negative result does *not* exclude pregnancy. It is always worthwhile to repeat a laboratory test when the result is unexpected. Tubal pregnancy is not uncommon and should always be considered if endometrial samples suggest gestational change without chorionic villi.

356. The answer is D. *(Robbins, 4/e. pp 1121–1125. Wilson, 12/e. pp 1630–1632.)* Over 95 percent of prostatic cancers are adenocarcinomas. In nearly 75 percent of cases adenocarcinoma of the prostate arises in the posterior lobe, usually in a subcapsular location. The lateral lobes are the next, much less frequent site. Nodular hyperplasia occurs in the periurethral region. When prostatic cancer is extracapsular or metastatic (commonly osteoblastic metastases to pelvis and lumbar vertebrae), serum tumor markers such as prostatic acid phosphatase (PAP) are detectable by standard assays. Tumor growth may be inhibited by estrogen therapy; it is not estrogen-dependent. Invasion of capsule, blood vessels, and perineural spaces is useful in diagnosis of well-differentiated tumor. Diagnosis may include needle biopsy or fine needle aspiration (80 percent accuracy).

357. The answer is C. *(Anderson, 9/e. pp 1667–1668.) Neisseria gonorrhoeae* is a very common bacterium that causes acute pelvic inflammatory disease with salpingitis in this country as a result of venereal infection. Tuboovarian abscesses may develop from this bacterium, as well as other bacteria, but these organisms are susceptible to penicillin therapy. In the presence of unresponsiveness to penicillin, consideration should be given to *Bacteroides* species, which are important anaerobic gram-negative bacilli and are generally refractory to penicillin. These anaerobic bacteria may produce serious infections if uncontrolled. Chlamydiae, while considered to be nongonococcal in origin, are nevertheless important agents in venereal transmission and often are contracted at the same time as *Neisseria* species. When the gonococcus is adequately treated with penicillin, and symptoms continue, there may have been concurrent infection with chlamydia that is not responsive to penicillin but is sensitive to tetracycline. Adenoviruses are responsible for keratoconjunctivitis, tracheobronchitis, pneumonia in children, acute gastroenteritis, and occasionally hemorrhagic cystitis, but are not ordinarily causative in pelvic inflammatory disease.

358. The answer is B. *(Anderson, 9/e. pp 808, 818–819.)* There are numerous causes of nephrotic syndrome (NS), including immune complex diseases, diabetes, amyloidosis, toxemia of pregnancy, and such circulating disturbances as bilateral renal vein thrombosis, but NS in small children (under 3 years of age) should suggest the possibility of the renal disease known as *minimal change* *nephropathy,* which is synonymous with *foot process disease,* or *nil disease.* This peculiar entity presents clinically as insidious nephrotic syndrome, characteristically occurring in younger children, but also seen in adults (rarely), with hypoalbuminemia, edema, hyperlipidemia, massive proteinuria, and lipiduria. The glomeruli are known for their rather normal appearance on light microscopy—at worst, there is mild and focal sclerosis. Electron microscopy is necessary for demonstrating characteristic attenuation and flattening of the foot processes of the podocytes attached to the Bowman's space side of the glomerular basement membrane. The podocytes may revert to normal (with steroid immunosuppressive therapy), or the foot-process attenuation may persist to some extent, in which case the proteinuria also persists. To date, no immune complex deposits or abnormalities of the glomerular basement membrane or mesangium have been demonstrated ultrastructurally.

359. The answer is D. *(Robbins, 4/e. pp 1150–1151.)* Cystic endometrial hyperplasia* refers to the abnormal growth of endometrium associated with either an absolute or a relative estrogen excess. These are common findings at the time of menopause and in conditions causing an absolute excess of estrogen—e.g., Stein-Leventhal syndrome, functioning granulosa and thecal cell ovarian tumors, and the exogenous administration of estrogenic substances. The microscopic findings in an endometrial biopsy are dominated by the marked dilatation of the endometrial glands, which gives the tissue section the appearance of Swiss cheese. The glands are lined by benign columnar epithelium that is nonsecretory.

360. The answer is D. *(Robbins, 4/e. pp 1012–1018.)* The unique structure and composition of the glomerular basement membrane and associated cells account for the formation of the plasma ultrafiltrate referred to as *urine.* The glomerular basement membrane is approximately 320 nm wide in the normal human with a central electron-dense lamina densa and electron-lucent lamina rara interna and externa with fenestrated endothelial cells immediately adjacent to the capillaries and the visceral epithelial cells (podocytes). Glomerular basement membrane is made up of collagen type 4, with laminen especially concentrated on both laminae rarae. Clustered also on both laminae rarae are polyanionic proteoglycans (especially heparan sulfate), which are thought to play a major role in the exclusion of albumin in the urinary filtrate by a mechanism of charge dependence restriction. This is based on the electronegative charge of the proteoglycans and the anionic charges of albumin. The mechanism is based on different isoelectric points. Thus it is felt that the glomerulus, because of these proteoglycans, may be able to discriminate materials passing through the glomerulus according to electronegative charge. Glomerular basement membrane does function by exclusion of materials based on size. Mesangial cells, by nature of their contractility, are thought to control intraglomerular blood flow under neurohormonal stimulation. Mesangial cells are not thought to function in filtration per se. The parietal cells lining the Bowman's membrane may function as a barrier but do not participate in the ultrafiltration. The fenestrated endothelial cells and podocytes are part of the filtering membranes but probably play a minor role compared with the glomerular polyanion barrier.

361. The answer is A. *(Robbins, 4/e. pp 1152–1153.)* The condition illustrated is a uterine leiomyoma (fibroid). This is an extremely common tumor occurring in up to 25 percent of women of reproductive age. The cause is unknown, but the growth is estrogen-dependent and for this reason the tumor may enlarge rapidly during pregnancy. If the tumor becomes very large, areas within it may undergo softening followed by liquefaction and cystic degeneration. Fibroids tend to regress in the postmenopausal period; with atrophy they become collagenous and calcification often occurs.

362. The answer is E. *(Anderson, 9/e. pp 379–382.)* Cytomegalic inclusion disease is diagnosed in the immunosuppressed or AIDS patient by finding large intranuclear inclusions surrounded by a clear halo in enlarged cells in urinary sediment, in sputum or bronchial lavage, in spinal fluid specimens, or in liver biopsy. Small intracytoplasmic inclusions may be found. Cytomegalovirus (CMV) is a DNA member of the herpesvirus group that causes disseminated disease, including interstitial pneumonitis in the debilitated or immunosuppressed adult. Disseminated infection with CMV in AIDS is associated with pneumonitis, hepatitis, idiopathic ulcerative colitis, encephalitis, and retinitis. Rising antibody titers may not be detectable for up to 4 weeks after primary infection and early diagnosis may be achieved by finding typical inclusion bodies in cytologic or biopsy specimens. However, the shell vial technique has revolutionized detection of CMV in cell culture with detection of early antigen in 24 h instead of 1 to 3 weeks.

363. The answer is E. *(Robbins, 4/e. pp 1012–1014.)* It has been recently shown that polyanionic molecules at sites on the luminal endothelial cells retard anions by electronegativity forces, aiding the transport of cationic proteins. They may greatly increase vascular permeability, especially in the renal glomerulus. The glomerular basement membrane contains the glycoprotein entactin, fibronectin, collagen type IV, laminen, and polyanionic proteoglycans (heparan sulfate) found at sites on both laminae rarae. The glomerular filtration barrier is made possible by these polyanions. The podocyte is attached to the lamina rara externa on the epithelial (urine filtrate) side of the glomerular basement membrane. Desmin is an intermediate filament protein found in fibroblasts and muscle cells. Bowman's capsule epithelial cells line the inner side of the glomerulus and are bathed in urinary ultrafiltrate. Fibronectin—a connective tissue protein formed by endothelial cells, fibroblasts, and macrophages—stabilizes endothelial cell attachments and functions in wound healing.

364. The answer is D. *(Robbins, 4/e. pp 1104–1105.)* The condition illustrated is acute orchitis. There is hemorrhage and inflammation in and between tubules with disruption of spermatogenesis. Bacteria are present in the tubules. Orchitis is somewhat less common than epididymitis and, when present, is usually due to extension of infection from the urinary tract via epididymal lymphatics or the vas deferens. Infection is rarely blood-borne. *E. coli* and *C. trachomatis* are the most common pathogens. Sequelae include tubular atrophy and excretory duct obstruction, both of which may cause sterility. Chronic infection may occur. Interstitial cells are more likely to survive or regenerate, so sexual function is often retained.

365. The answer is D. *(Graves, N Engl J Med 312:338, 1985.)* Measuring acid phosphatase intracellularly by the immunohistochemical method for in situ cells as in a needle biopsy is specific for prostate source, as is the same determination for prostatic specific antigen. Circulating plasma levels of prostatic acid phosphatase are elevated in circumstances of metastatic prostate adenocarcinoma. Alkaline phosphatases are found within the liver, placenta, and bone. Measurement of a recently described protein in semen is highly specific for seminal fluid, and the detection of the presence of p30 antigen in vaginal fluid is conclusive evidence that coitus has taken place. The test is an ELISA determination.

366. The answer is B. *(Robbins, 4/e. pp 1075–1077.)* Renal cell carcinoma (renal adenocarcinoma) accounts for 85 percent of primary renal tumors and usually occurs in the sixth decade, although sometimes at a much younger age. These tumors may produce hormones or hormonelike substances, for example, renin (hypertension), glucocorticoids (Cushing's syndrome), and gonadotropins (feminization and masculinization). More frequently, though in only 5 to 10 percent of patients, polycythemia or erythrocytosis occurs owing to production of erythropoietin. Renal cell carcinoma is not associated with tuberous sclerosis in which the common renal lesion is angiomyolipoma (hamartoma). It is associated with the von Hippel–Lindau syndrome in which many patients develop bilateral renal cell carcinomas. Translocations between chromosomes 3 and 8 and 3 and 11 have been found in some cases of familial renal cancer and in a few sporadic cases. Hematuria is often the first symptom but often occurs late, after invasion of the renal vein or widespread metastases frequently to lung, bone, or brain. Renal cell carcinoma is predominantly of clear cell type with intracytoplasmic glycogen and lipid, but less often granular cells with numerous mitochondria or spindle cells occur. Diagnosis requires IVP, CT, and ultrasound to differentiate benign cysts, as well as percutaneous needle aspiration for cytology.

367. The answer is D. *(Robbins, 4/e. p 1138.)* Neoplasms of the vagina are rare, but of these squamous cell carcinoma is the most common. Vaginal clear cell adenocarcinoma occurs occasionally (1 or less per 1000) in girls in their late teens whose mothers had received diethylstilbestrol during pregnancy. In about one-third of cases, such cancers arise in the cervix. More frequently, in about half of the population at risk, small glandular or microcystic lesions appear in the mucosa—vaginal adenosis. These benign lesions appear as red, velvety foci and are lined by mucus-secreting or ciliated columnar cells. From these areas in the rarer clear cell adenocarcinoma arises. Sarcoma botryoides, producing soft polypoid grapelike masses, is another rare primary vaginal cancer found usually in infants and children under age 5. It is a rhabdomyosarcoma that can also occur in the urinary bladder.

368–371. The answers are: 368-B, 369-C, 370-D, 371-E. *(Robbins, 4/e. pp 1031–1044. Rose, 2/e. pp 223–224.)* Membranoproliferative glomerulonephritis occurs in two types. Type I, which is associated with nephrotic syndrome, is driven by immune complexes; type II is associated with hematuria and chronic renal failure and, in addition to immune complexes, involves alternate complement activation. In either type there is mesangial proliferation accompanied by thickening of the glomerular basement membranes, and a special finding that often supports the diagnosis of membranoproliferative glomerulonephritis is the presence of actual splitting of the glomerular basement membranes. In type I there are subendothelial deposits of IgG, C3, C1, and C4. In type II there are dense deposits of C3 (dense-deposit disease) with or without IgG and no C1.

Membranous glomerulonephritis, rather than being driven by an immune complex, is antibody-mediated and results in diffuse thickening of glomerular capillary walls by subepithelial deposits of IgG and C3 in a diffuse involvement of the glomeruli. These deposits are seen by fluorescence as granular deposits. Membranous glomerulonephritis is also associated with the nephrotic syndrome.

In PSGN the light microscope histology consists of diffuse endothelial and mesangial cell proliferation with neutrophil infiltration, so that narrowing of capillary lumens and enlargement of the glomerular tuft to fill Bowman's space occur. Electron microscopy reveals the mesangial deposits and hump-shaped subepithelial deposits in peripheral capillary loops that are so characteristic of PSGN. Immunofluorescence shows granular deposits containing IgG, C3, and often fibrin in glomerular capillary walls and mesangium.

Goodpasture's syndrome is an acute, serious disease often heralded by pulmonary hemorrhages and remarkable hemoptysis accompanied by acute glomerulonephritis that often is of the rapidly progressive form. Antiglomerular basement membrane antibodies are seen in Goodpasture's syndrome, which result in IgG linear deposits along the glomerular basement membranes. Also seen are marked and dramatic formations of epithelial cell crescents accompanied by infiltrates of monocytes and neutrophils with fibrin deposition and necrosis of epithelial and endothelial cells. There is no accompanying fragmentation of glomerular basement membranes as there is in membranoproliferative glomerulonephritis.

Hyalinized glomeruli may be seen in any terminal glomerulonephritis (GN) but are best seen in chronic renal failure caused by chronic GN.

372–376. The answers are: 372-D, 373-A, 374-B, 375-A, 376-C. *(Robbins, 4/e. pp 1174–1178.)* The trophoblastic tumors include the benign hydatidiform mole, the invasive mole (chorioadenoma destruens), and choriocarcinoma. Hydatidiform mole occurs in the U.S. in about 1 in 2000 pregnancies. Both hydatidiform mole and choriocarcinoma produce high levels of human chorionic gonadotropin (hCG); the levels are extremely high in choriocarcinoma unless considerable tumor necrosis is present. Alpha-fetoprotein is not produced by trophoblastic tumors, in contrast to embryonal carcinoma and teratomas, which both may produce alpha-fetoprotein and human chorionic gonadotropin simultaneously. Choriocarcinoma shows the following incidence: 50 percent arise in moles, 25 percent follow abortion, and about 22 percent arise in normal pregnancy; the remainder originate in ectopic pregnancies and extragenital and genital teratomas, including teratoma of the testis. The cure rate for choriocarcinoma is very high (up to 80 percent) with chemotherapy of methotrexate and actinomycin.

377–380. The answers are: 377-C, 378-B, 379-A, 380-B. *(Robbins, 4/e. pp 1036–1038.)* Minimal change disease (MCD), or lipoid nephrosis, is the most common cause of the nephrotic syndrome in children (65 percent of cases; 10 to 20 percent of adult cases). In MCD loss or flattening of foot processes of epithelial cells occurs, but immunofluorescence shows no immunoglobulin or complement deposits. Renal biopsy may be required to differentiate early MCD from early membranous glomerulonephritis (MGN), but subepithelial immunoglobulin deposits are found in MGN and developed cases show diffuse thickening of the glomerular capillary wall. Glomeruli in MCD appear virtually normal by light microscopy. Rapid response to steroid therapy and excellent long-term prognosis characterize MCD.

Focal segmental glomerulosclerosis (FSG) accounts for about 10 to 15 percent of cases of nephrotic syndrome in both children and adults. The characteristic change in some glomeruli (focal) consists of areas of mesangial sclerosis with collapse of capillary loops spreading out from the central tuft. Other changes may include occlusion of capillary lumina by hyaline protein deposits (hyalinosis). Immunofluorescence shows IgM and C3, mostly in sclerotic mesangial areas. The electron-microscopic changes are mesangial sclerosis in affected glomeruli and fusion of foot processes in all glomeruli—changes similar to those seen in MCD. Most cases of FSG are idiopathic, but the nephrotic syndrome and FSG are found in more than 10 percent of patients with AIDS, as well as in chronic intravenous heroin users. Since T-cell function in AIDS is so abnormal, release of a toxic lymphokine could be responsible for the glomerular injury. Response to steroid therapy is poor and more than 50 percent of the patients die, or have persistent disease, within 10 years of diagnosis.

381–384. The answers are: 381-B, 382-D, 383-A, 384-E. *(Robbins, 4/e. pp 857–858, 1158–1159, 1163–1164, 1167–1170.)* The Krukenberg tumor is usually a bilateral ovarian tumor. It practically always metastasizes from the gastrointestinal tract and most frequently arises from a gastric adenocarcinoma. Histologically, there is diffuse infiltration of mucinous signet-ring cells.

The ovarian fibroma is a relatively common, benign ovarian tumor (about 4 percent of all types) that may be accompanied by ascites in about 40 percent of all cases. Less common is pleural effusion, often right-sided. The combination of ovarian fibroma, ascites, and hydrothorax is known as Meigs' syndrome. Rarely, the basal cell nevus syndrome is associated.

The granulosa-theca cell tumors are sex cord–stromal in origin and account for 5 percent of all ovarian tumors. They range from almost pure granulosa cell tumors to pure thecomas. These tumors may occur at any age, but about two-thirds occur in postmenopausal women and, because of estrogen production, may be associated with endometrial hyperplasia, endometrial carcinoma, or cystic breast disease. Tumors with a large thecal component may cause precocious sexual development in prepubertal girls. Granulosa-theca cell tumors are potentially malignant (5 to 25 percent), but pure thecomas are not.

Endometrioid tumors are approximately 20 percent of all ovarian cancers; they may be carcinomas, borderline lesions, or benign. Up to 30 percent of the carcinomas are associated with endometrial carcinoma or endometriosis. They are solid and cystic tumors containing tubular glands similar to those of benign or malignant endometrium. About 40 percent are bilateral and the 5-year survival rate is 40 to 50 percent.

Brenner tumors, 2 percent of ovarian neoplasms, are usually benign, solid, often small, unilateral tumors. Their dense, fibrous stroma has nests of transitional cells like urothelium.

385–388. The answers are: 385-B, 386-C, 387-D, 388-A. *(Robbins, 4/e. pp 1058–1059, 1062–1068, 1172–1174.)* Benign nephrosclerosis, renal disease occurring in benign hypertension, is characterized by hyaline arteriolosclerosis with thickened hyalinized arteriolar walls and narrowed lumina. Fibroelastic hyperplasia occurs in the larger muscular arteries. Small kidneys with granular surfaces often result because of ischemic atrophy of nephrons.

Renal arteriolar changes in malignant nephrosclerosis (malignant hypertension) include fibrinoid necrosis of arterioles (necrotizing arteriolitis), hyperplastic arteriolosclerosis (onion-skinning), necrotizing glomerulitis, and often a thrombotic microangiopathy. The clinical course is often downhill with only 50 percent of patients surviving 5 years; marked proteinuria, hematuria, cardiovascular problems, and finally renal failure contribute to death. The disease is often associated with accelerated preexisting benign essential hypertension, chronic renal disease (glomerulonephritis), or scleroderma.

Preeclampsia is characterized by hypertension, proteinuria, and edema that begins after 20 weeks of gestation but is obvious clinically after 32 weeks. Most common in the last trimester of a first pregnancy, it occurs in about 6 percent of all pregnancies. It may progress to eclampsia with convulsions and coma. Renal involvement involves the glomeruli with narrowing or obliteration of capillary lumens due to swelling of endothelial and mesangial cells (glomerular endotheliosis). Electron microscopy shows widening of the subendothelial region between basement membrane and endothelial cell by electron-lucent and dense material (fibrin), this change being similar to that in HUS. Pathogenesis includes placental ischemia with decreased production of vasodilator prostaglandins (PGI_2, PGE_2) and increased release of vasoconstrictors.

Analgesic abuse nephropathy (analgesic nephritis) occurs because of excessive intake of *mixtures* of aspirin and phenacetin. It requires the synergistic action of these drugs and cases due to aspirin, or phenacetin, or acetaminophen alone are rare. Analgesic abuse nephropathy eventually results in papillary necrosis (necrotizing papillitis) with secondary chronic tubulointerstitial nephritis. Clinical findings include sterile pyuria, anemia, GI symptoms, urinary tract infections, and hypertension. Chronic renal failure may occur, but drug withdrawal often stabilizes kidney function. There is, however, an increased incidence of urothelial carcinoma of the renal pelvis.

Nervous System

DIRECTIONS: Each question below contains five suggested responses. Select the **one best** response to each question.

389. Which of the following conditions is the most frequent cause of intracerebral hemorrhage?

(A) Ruptured aneurysm
(B) Trauma
(C) Blood dyscrasias
(D) Angiomas
(E) Hypertensive vascular disease

390. A 9-year-old boy who had been suffering from a gait disturbance for several weeks was found to have a posterior fossa mass on CT scan. The most likely cause for these findings is

(A) a berry aneurysm
(B) astrocytoma
(C) medulloblastoma
(D) oligodendroglioma
(E) pseudotumor cerebri

391. Tuberculous leptomeningitis is

(A) associated with smooth-walled cavities in the brain
(B) often associated with subdural effusion
(C) often a result of vertebral infection
(D) usually located over the cerebral convexities
(E) often part of miliary infection in children

392. A 55-year-old woman is suspected of having a brain tumor because of the onset of seizure activity. Computerized tomograms (CT scans) and skull x-rays demonstrate a mass in the right cerebral hemisphere that is markedly calcific. A high index of suspicion should exist for

(A) oligodendroglioma
(B) astrocytoma
(C) cerebral lymphoma
(D) metastatic carcinoma
(E) brown tumor

393. Retinoblastoma, the most common intraocular tumor of children, is associated with all the following EXCEPT

(A) occurrence in both familial and sporadic patterns
(B) unilateral and unifocal sporadic tumors
(C) inactivation of cancer suppressor genes
(D) poor prognosis even with treatment
(E) frequent histologic occurrence of rosettes

394. All the following have been commonly associated with pyogenic brain abscesses EXCEPT

(A) congenital heart disease
(B) sinusitis
(C) lung abscess
(D) liver abscess
(E) mastoiditis

395. Subdural hematomas occur most frequently in the

(A) supracerebellar region
(B) infracerebellar region
(C) cerebellopontine angle
(D) pituitary region
(E) cerebral hemisphere convexities

396. Select the disorder below that has the most clinicopathologic features in common with postvaccinal encephalomyelitis.

(A) Metachromatic leukodystrophy
(B) Multifocal leukoencephalopathy
(C) Guillain-Barré syndrome
(D) Hypoxic encephalopathy
(E) Hypertensive encephalopathy

397. Which of the following tumors is characterized by pseudopalisading, necrosis, endoneurial proliferation, hypercellularity, and atypical nuclei?

(A) Schwannoma
(B) Medulloblastoma
(C) Oligodendroglioma
(D) Glioblastoma multiforme
(E) Ependymoma

398. A young patient is found comatose in an automobile with the windows up and the engine running. Death ensues within 3 days and an autopsy is performed. Sections through the brain would show

(A) subdural hematoma
(B) epidural hematoma
(C) basilar hemorrhage
(D) brainstem hemorrhages
(E) hemorrhages of the lenticular nuclei

399. All the following statements apply to ependymomas EXCEPT that

(A) they are the most common type of intraspinal glioma
(B) they are the most common primary brain tumor in children
(C) patients may present with headache and papilledema
(D) they may require differentiation from choroid plexus papilloma
(E) histologic sections display rosettes

400. The most frequent of all the following intracranial tumors in adults is

(A) ependymoma
(B) medulloblastoma
(C) meningioma
(D) glioma
(E) metastasis

401. Creutzfeldt-Jakob disease displays all the following characteristics EXCEPT

(A) spongiform encephalopathy
(B) rapidly progressive dementia
(C) worldwide incidence of 1 case per 100,000 population
(D) absence of an inflammatory infiltrate
(E) inactivation by hypochlorite solution

402. The form of motor neuron disease in which there is weakness and atrophy of muscles, without corticospinal tract dysfunction, is known as

(A) amyotrophic lateral sclerosis
(B) progressive muscular atrophy
(C) Werdnig-Hoffmann syndrome
(D) primary lateral sclerosis
(E) Charcot-Marie-Tooth disease

403. Cerebral neuroblastomas are known to

(A) be fairly common brain tumors
(B) be most common in intrauterine life
(C) usually form mature ganglion cells
(D) elaborate catecholamines rarely
(E) usually form extraneural metastases

404. True statements about meningiomas include all the following EXCEPT

(A) they are more common in women
(B) they constitute 15 to 20 percent of primary brain tumors
(C) they usually display rapid growth
(D) they arise from arachnoid cap cells
(E) they may be multiple

405. Cerebral embolism occurs frequently in association with all the following conditions EXCEPT

(A) cardiac mural thrombi
(B) left-sided endocarditis
(C) right-sided endocarditis
(D) cardiac catheterization
(E) prosthetic cardiac valves

406. Transection of a peripheral nerve will result in all the following EXCEPT

(A) dissolution of the Nissl substance in the nerve cell body
(B) degeneration of the nerve fiber distal to the cut
(C) proliferation of the Schwann sheath from the proximal nerve segment
(D) loss of the entire Schwann sheath proximal to the cut
(E) degeneration of the axons from 1 to 3 nodes of Ranvier proximal to the cut

407. Lesions associated with acquired immunodeficiency syndrome (AIDS) include all the following EXCEPT

(A) abscess of brain
(B) primary malignant lymphoma of brain
(C) subacute encephalitis with multinucleate cells
(D) progressive multifocal leukoencephalopathy
(E) aseptic meningitis

408. The major features of tuberous sclerosis include all the following EXCEPT

(A) mental retardation and seizures
(B) renal angiomyolipomas
(C) hypoplasia of the cerebellar vermis
(D) pancreatic cysts and cardiac rhabdomyomas
(E) skin angiofibromas (adenoma sebaceum)

409. Intracerebral calcification is associated with all the following EXCEPT

(A) glioblastoma multiforme
(B) tuberous sclerosis
(C) oligodendroglioma
(D) craniopharyngioma
(E) hypoparathyroidism

410. True statements regarding neuroglial cells include all the following EXCEPT

(A) they include astrocytes
(B) they include oligodendrocytes
(C) they include ependymal cells and microglial cells
(D) all function to shelter and maintain neurons
(E) all function as macrophages, when activated

411. A known alcoholic is brought to the emergency room following an altercation in a local bar. The intern observes respiratory irregularity, coma, and papilledema. Emergency surgery is planned in order to prevent all the following EXCEPT

(A) brainstem herniation
(B) cerebellar herniation
(C) Duret hemorrhages
(D) ruptured aneurysm
(E) death of the patient

412. True statements about classic neurofibromatosis (von Recklinghausen's disease) include all the following EXCEPT

(A) axillary freckling is characteristic
(B) hamartomas of the iris are very common
(C) hemangioblastomas of the brain are associated
(D) acoustic neuroma is associated
(E) pheochromocytomas and meningiomas are associated

413. Clinicopathologic features of amyotrophic lateral sclerosis (ALS) include all the following EXCEPT

(A) degeneration in the pyramidal motor system
(B) sensory loss secondary to involvement of dorsal nerve roots
(C) loss of anterior horn neurons
(D) loss of myelinated fibers in corticospinal tracts
(E) dysphagia

414. All the following tumors may be found arising within the pineal gland EXCEPT

(A) teratoma
(B) pineoblastoma
(C) embryonal carcinoma
(D) choriocarcinoma
(E) craniopharyngioma

415. Diseases that are classified as slow viral infections or unconventional agent (spongiform) encephalopathies include all the following EXCEPT

(A) Reye's syndrome
(B) subacute sclerosing panencephalitis
(C) Creutzfeldt-Jakob disease
(D) progressive multifocal leukoencephalopathy
(E) kuru

416. Syringomyelia is characterized by all the following EXCEPT

(A) segmental loss of pain and temperature sensation
(B) segmental loss of touch sensation
(C) loss of tissue (cavitation) within the cervical spinal cord
(D) small muscle atrophy of the hands
(E) kyphoscoliosis

417. In subacute combined degeneration (SCD) there is

(A) association with hemolytic anemia
(B) usually involvement of gray matter of the spinal cord
(C) usually no motor impairment
(D) failure of the enzyme methylmalonic CoA mutase
(E) dermatitis, enteritis, and dementia

418. All the following are features of tabes dorsalis EXCEPT

(A) bilateral degeneration of dorsal nerve roots
(B) a positive Romberg sign
(C) severe impairment of vibratory sense
(D) progressive sensitivity to pain
(E) Argyll Robertson pupils

419. The lesion shown in the photomicrograph below was removed from a patient's nasal cavity. With no age given and at this low magnification, the most likely diagnosis is

(A) adenocarcinoma
(B) nasal glioma
(C) olfactory neuroblastoma
(D) nasopharyngeal angiofibroma
(E) multiple myeloma

420. Alzheimer's disease is characterized by all the following EXCEPT

(A) cerebral atrophy in superior temporal and frontal lobes
(B) neuritic or senile plaques
(C) amyloid β-protein deposits
(D) Lewy bodies
(E) granulovacuolar degeneration

DIRECTIONS: Each group of questions below consists of lettered headings followed by a set of numbered items. For each numbered item select the **one** lettered heading with which it is **most** closely associated. Each lettered heading may be used **once, more than once, or not at all.**

Questions 421–425

For each of the conditions below, choose the most appropriate description.

    (A) Herniation of the meninges alone
    (B) Herniation of meninges and brain parenchyma
    (C) Developmental bone defect
    (D) Herniation of meninges and a portion of the spinal cord
    (E) Herniation at the roof of the mouth

421. Cranium bifidum

422. Meningocele

423. Meningoencephalocele

424. Spina bifida

425. Meningomyelocele

Questions 426–432

For each disease, choose the sign with which it is most likely to be associated.

    (A) Accumulation of GM_2 ganglioside
    (B) Genetic defect on chromosome 21
    (C) Primary CNS demyelination
    (D) Abnormal or defective myelin metabolism
    (E) Genetic defect on chromosome 4

426. Familial Alzheimer's disease

427. Huntington's disease

428. Multiple sclerosis

429. Krabbe's disease

430. Tay-Sachs disease

431. Metachromatic leukodystrophy

432. Postinfectious encephalomyelitis

Questions 433–439

For each disease, choose the sign with which it is most likely to be associated.

(A) Neurofibrillary tangles
(B) Cowdry A intranuclear inclusions
(C) Optic nerve demyelination
(D) Hepatolenticular degeneration
(E) Verocay bodies
(F) Lewy bodies

433. Postencephalitic parkinsonism

434. Idiopathic parkinsonism

435. Herpes simplex encephalitis

436. Wilson's disease

437. Pick's disease

438. Schwannoma

439. Devic's syndrome

Nervous System
Answers

389. The answer is E. *(Robbins, 4/e. pp 1405–1406.)* Hypertension is 10 to 20 times more frequent than all the other causes of intracerebral hemorrhage and is also the most common cause of death from cerebrovascular disease. Major sites of hemorrhage are the putamen (more than 50 percent); the cortex and subcortex (15 percent); and the thalamus, the pons, and the cerebellum (each approximately 10 percent). Hypertensive hemorrhage shows a predilection for the distribution of the lenticulostriate arteries with small (lacunar) hemorrhages, or large hemorrhages obliterating the corpus striatum, including the putamen and internal capsule. It is possible that development of microaneurysms (Charcot-Bouchard aneurysms) with subsequent rupture is a precipitating factor.

390. The answer is C. *(Robbins, 4/e. pp 1419–1420.)* Astrocytomas are not at all uncommon in the younger age group, but when a child presents with clinical symptoms pointing to the intracranial posterior fossa, a cerebellar medulloblastoma should be suspected, especially if the child has no prior history of leukemia or neuroblastoma. Medulloblastomas occur predominantly in childhood and usually arise in the midline of the cerebellum (the vermis). They do occur (less commonly) in adults, in whom they are more apt to arise in the cerebellar hemispheres in a lateral position. They grow by local invasive growth and may block cerebrospinal fluid circulation (CSF block) by compression of the fourth ventricle. Recent aggressive treatment with the combined modalities of excision, radiotherapy, and chemotherapy have improved survival.

391. The answer is E. *(Anderson, 9/e. pp 2154–2156.)* Smooth-walled cavities in the gray matter are frequent with cryptococcal meningitis, while in tuberculous meningitis solid granulomas may occur in meninges or brain. Subdural effusion is common in *Haemophilus influenzae* meningitis, a common cause of meningitis in early childhood, but is rare in tuberculosis where the exudate is prominent at the base of the brain. Tuberculous infection rarely extends from vertebra to epidural and subdural spaces. In adults it is usually associated with lung disease and in young children with generalized miliary infection. *Mycobacterium tuberculosis* is a strict aerobe and cerebrospinal fluid cultures should never commence with culture tubes upright or horizontal.

392.   The answer is A. *(Robbins, 4/e. pp 1416–1417.)* Although several lesions within the brain may be associated with dystrophic or metaplastic calcification, the presence of a calcified tumorlike mass lesion in the cerebral hemispheres should arouse suspicion of oligodendroglioma. Oligodendrogliomas are often slow-growing gliomas composed of round cells with clear cytoplasm ("fried-egg appearance"); they generally occur in the fourth and fifth decades of life. However, some oligodendrogliomas do proliferate in a rapid and aggressive fashion and may be associated with a malignant astrocytoma component. The brown tumor associated with hypercalcemia of hyperparathyroidism is associated with osteitis fibrosa cystica of bone. Some metastatic carcinomas may show microcalcifications in the form of psammoma bodies, as do some meningiomas. Papillary carcinomas of the thyroid and ovary are the best examples of such lesions, but the calcifications found in papillary carcinomas are rarely of the degree and magnitude of those found in some oligodendrogliomas.

393.   The answer is D. *(Robbins, 4/e. pp 289–291, 1462–1463.)* Familial cases of retinoblastoma are frequently multiple and bilateral, although like all the sporadic, nonheritable tumors they can also be unifocal and unilateral. Histologically, rosettes of various types are frequent (similar to neuroblastoma and medulloblastoma). There is a good prognosis with early detection and treatment; spontaneous regression occurs rarely. Retinoblastoma belongs to a group of cancers (osteosarcoma, Wilms' tumor, meningioma, rhabdomyosarcoma, uveal melanoma) in which the normal cancer suppressor gene (antioncogene) is inactivated or lost, with resultant malignant change. Retinoblastoma and osteosarcoma arise after loss of the same genetic locus—hereditary mutation in the q14 band of chromosome 13. Probably the normal 13 q14 locus is a suppressor gene.

394.   The answer is D. *(Anderson, 9/e. p 2158.)* Pyogenic brain abscesses may have a number of possible sources, but the origin can often be determined from the location and number of abscesses in the brain parenchyma. Isolated lesions in the frontal lobes often arise from extension of sinus infections. In the temporal lobe or cerebellum, an isolated lesion may have the middle ear or mastoid as the primary site. Multiple lesions, especially in the superior aspects of the cerebrum, are seen with hematogenous dissemination, often from lung infection or in association with the lesions of congenital heart disease.

395.   The answer is E. *(Anderson, 9/e. pp 2187–2188.)* When blood enters the potential space between the arachnoid and dura, a subdural hematoma forms.

Subdural hematomas are most commonly located over the cerebral hemisphere convexities. The traditional explanation for the formation of subdural hematomas has been tearing of the bridging veins that pass from the cortical surface to the superior sagittal sinus. Blood may also leak from lacerated cortical vessels or arachnoidal vessels ruptured by a meningeal tear.

396. The answer is C. *(Robbins, 4/e. pp 315, 1444.)* Guillain-Barré (GB) syndrome (acute inflammatory polyradiculoneuropathy) is similar to postinfectious (or postvaccinal) encephalomyelitis in that both cause a process of demyelination and show perivascular infiltrates of lymphoid cells (in the brain and brainstem in encephalomyelitis and in the craniospinal nerve, roots, and ganglia in GB syndrome). In addition, the anterior horn cells in GB syndrome may be degenerative. GB syndrome manifests clinically as lower limb weakness and paralysis with varying sensory disturbances, such as hypesthesia of the lower limbs. The disease may progress to involvement of the musculature of the upper body, including the muscles of respiration, which can lead to respiratory arrest in the absence of mechanical ventilatory assistance. GB syndrome was identified in some persons who were vaccinated with influenza vaccines during the late 1970s.

397. The answer is D. *(Robbins, 4/e. pp 1414–1417, 1445–1446.)* Schwannomas generally appear as extremely cellular, spindle cell neoplasms, sometimes with metaplastic elements of bone, cartilage, and skeletal muscle. Medulloblastomas occur exclusively in the cerebellum and microscopically are highly cellular with uniform nuclei, scant cytoplasm, and, in about one-third of cases, rosette formation centered by neurofibrillary material. Oligodendrogliomas, which are marked by foci of calcification in 70 percent of cases, commonly show a pattern of uniform cellularity and are composed of round cells with small dark nuclei, clear cytoplasm, and a clearly defined cell membrane. Ependymomas are distinguished by ependymal rosettes, which are ductlike structures with a central lumen around which columnar tumor cells are arranged in a concentric fashion.

398. The answer is E. *(Anderson, 9/e. pp 220–222.)* Incomplete combustion of any carbon fuel will lead to accumulation of carbon monoxide gases. Oxygen deprivation results from the formation of carboxyhemoglobin, which displaces the normal oxyhemoglobin and interferes with oxygen exchange. In addition to small petechial hemorrhages of serosa and white matter of the cerebral hemispheres, patients who have lived for several days following exposure will have gross lesions in the brain that consist of bilateral hemorrhage and necrosis of the globus pallidus and hippocampus.

399. The answer is B. *(Robbins, 4/e. pp 1417–1418.)* Astrocytomas are the most common type of primary brain tumor in children and occur mainly in the cerebellum. Ependymomas often occur in childhood and adolescence but have been noted at all ages. They form more than 60 percent of intraspinal gliomas, but only about 5 percent of intracranial gliomas. Hydrocephalus can be a complication of intraventricular ependymoma. The papillary intraventricular ependymoma is similar grossly to the choroid plexus papilloma. Microscopically, the diagnostic rosette and pseudorosette formations are seen in the ependymoma, with tumor cells arranged around a central space (rosette) or around a blood vessel (pseudorosette). Blepharoplasts, the basal bodies of cilia, are pathognomonic if present.

400. The answer is D. *(Robbins, 4/e. pp 1414–1422.)* Gliomas are the most frequent intracranial tumors of adults; they constitute 40 to 50 percent of such tumors, with glioblastoma multiforme making up 25 to 30 percent. Gliomas at the opposite end of the spectrum include ependymoma and oligodendroglioma, each constituting only 2 to 3 percent. Medulloblastoma also forms 2 to 3 percent of intracranial tumors in adults. Astrocytomas have an 8 to 12 percent and meningiomas a 12 to 15 percent intracranial incidence. Metastatic tumors have an intracranial incidence of 25 to 30 percent; metastatic carcinoma (lung, breast, kidney, GI) and melanoma are predominant. Metastases are often multiple and demarcated from surrounding brain tissue.

401. The answer is C. *(Robbins, 4/e. pp 1400–1401.)* In Creutzfeldt-Jakob disease there is a spongiform change in the cortical gray matter and, sometimes, the basal ganglia are affected. There is little, or no, gross atrophy of the brain and no inflammatory response in brain tissue. The disease is similar to kuru in humans and scrapie in sheep and goats. Rapidly progressive dementia occurs. Worldwide incidence is about one case per million population. The disease is caused by transmissible agents, or prions, which are proteinaceous infective particles, resistant to formalin and ionizing radiation, but inactivated by autoclaving, hypochlorite solutions (bleach), and alcoholic iodine.

402. The answer is B. *(Robbins, 4/e. pp 1432–1433.)* Motor neuron disease is a progressive disorder of the motor neurons in the cerebral cortex, brainstem, and spinal cord and occurs in different forms, depending on the involvement of one or more of these anatomic sites. In progressive muscular atrophy, there is predominant involvement of anterior horn cells, with remittent weakness and atrophy of muscles but no evidence of the corticospinal tract dysfunction that is a finding in amyotrophic lateral sclerosis. However, the basic pathologic processes of these two diseases are similar.

403. The answer is D. *(Robbins, 4/e. pp 1266, 1418.)* The cerebral neuroblastoma is a rare primary malignant brain tumor, usually located in the cerebral hemispheres, and most common during the first 10 years of life. The neuroblastoma is, of course, more frequent in the adrenal medulla, with about 50 percent of neuroblastomas originating in the adrenal and most of the remainder in association with the sympathetic chain. In the cerebral neuroblastoma occasional maturation toward ganglion cells occurs, as in medulloblastoma and in the neuroblastoma of the adrenal medulla, and catecholamines are rarely elaborated, in contrast to the adrenal neuroblastoma. Dissemination of the cerebral neuroblastoma may occur by way of the CSF, as in medulloblastoma. Rare extraneural metastases may develop. Histologically, rosettes and pseudorosettes may be found, as in medulloblastoma and adrenal neuroblastoma.

404. The answer is C. *(Robbins, 4/e. pp 1420–1421.)* Meningiomas arise from arachnoid villi of brain or spinal cord and have a female:male ratio of 3:2. Although they are usually tumors of middle or later life, a small number occur in persons 20 to 40 years of age. They commonly arise along the venous sinuses (parasagittal, sphenoid wings, and olfactory groove). Although benign and usually slow-growing, some meningiomas have sex hormone receptors and rapid growth in pregnancy occurs occasionally. The rare malignant meningioma may invade or even metastasize. Histologically, syncytial, transitional, and fibroblastic forms occur; psammoma bodies are found, particularly in the transitional pattern. The cut surface often has a whorled appearance. Meningioma is usually solitary, but multiple meningiomas occur, especially in classic neurofibromatosis. Orbital meningiomas (female:male ratio of 5:1) may cause unilateral exophthalmos and often occur in patients under 20 years of age.

405. The answer is C. *(Wilson, 12/e. pp 1995–1996.)* Cerebral embolism is probably the most common cause of stroke and most cerebral emboli arise in the heart. Myocardial infarction with mural thrombi, atrial fibrillation thrombi, and left-sided bacterial endocarditis are frequent sources, but in right-sided bacterial endocarditis (drug addicts, patients with gonococcal endocarditis or ventricular septal defect) emboli to organs other than the lungs are very rare, except in paradoxical embolism of septal defect. Endocarditis must be excluded when cerebral embolism is suspected. Thromboembolism from prosthetic heart valves has not been unusual. Cardiac catheterization and other invasive procedures involving an atherosclerotic aorta or femoral or iliac arteries may cause atheroemboli (cholesterol emboli) with resultant small infarcts of brain, kidney, gut, skin, or other organs. At least 35 to 40 percent of all strokes are embolic, and emboli are the predominant cause of infarction in the area supplied by the middle cerebral artery.

406. The answer is D. *(Robbins, 4/e. pp 1442–1443.)* The axonal reaction that occurs when a peripheral nerve is cut includes a number of striking changes. In the cell body, swelling and dissolution of the Nissl substance are apparent within 24 to 48 h after transection. The axon and covering myelin or Schwann sheath distal to the lesion first degenerate and undergo resorption. In addition, the axis cylinder and Schwann sheath degenerate proximal to the cut over the distance of a few nodal segments. Regeneration occurs when the Schwann cells proliferate from the proximal portion to form a hollow myelin sheath through which the axons grow again.

407. The answer is A. *(Anderson, 9/e. pp 2163–2164. Robbins, 4/e. pp 1398–1399.)* AIDS presents a major defect of the cell-mediated immune system, occurrence of many opportunistic infections, and development of unusual tumors including Kaposi's sarcoma, cloacogenic carcinoma, and malignant lymphoma often involving head and neck regions and, occasionally, limited to the central nervous system or the liver. The neoplasm, often of large-cell type, is comparable to lymphoma in immunosuppressed renal-transplant patients. Formerly, it was called *microglioma*. Progressive multifocal leukoencephalopathy (PML) is an opportunistic viral infection of the central nervous system characterized by multiple foci of demyelination. It affects patients with altered immunologic states, such as lymphoproliferative disorders, and has been reported in patients with AIDS. Etiologic agents are the papovaviruses JC and SV 40 (-PML). Subacute encephalitis with multinucleate, often giant, cells is considered pathognomonic of HIV-1 encephalitis. It occurs in cerebral white matter and cord, and HIV-1 has been found in its macrophages and multinucleate cells. The AIDS dementia complex correlates with this lesion. An aseptic meningitis similar to viral meningitis occurs in 10 percent of AIDS patients and HIV has been isolated from CSF in some of these.

408. The answer is C. *(Robbins, 4/e. p 1441.)* Severe hypoplasia or absence of the cerebellar vermis occurs in Dandy-Walker malformation. There is a cystic distention of the roof of the fourth ventricle, which bulges posteriorly; hydrocephalus with dilated ventricles; and possibly agenesis of the corpus callosum. Tuberous sclerosis is one of the phakomatoses, which also include neurofibromatosis and von Hippel–Lindau disease; these are familial, progressive disorders with CNS, systemic, and skin manifestations. Tuberous sclerosis, an autosomal dominant disease of variable penetrance, may show characteristic brain lesions: firm, white nodules, or tubers, in the cortex and subependymal nodules of gliosis protruding into the ventricles ("candle drippings"). Microscopically, these subependymal lesions show large, multinucleate, bizarre astrocytes and may eventually form infiltrating astrocytomas. Major early signs in tuberous sclerosis include a triad of seizures, mental retardation, and congenital white spots or macules (leukoderma), which are found in all cases by the age of 2 years. Facial angiofibromata (adenoma sebaceum) are almost pathognomonic but may not appear until 3 to 4 years of age, so white macules are a better sign.

409. The answer is A. *(Robbins, 4/e. pp 1213, 1247, 1414–1417, 1441.)* Glioblastoma multiforme is a rapidly growing cerebral tumor in which calcification does not develop, but in which necrosis and hemorrhage are frequent. Both oligodendroglioma and craniopharyngioma show fairly frequent calcification; oligodendroglioma is often located in the frontal lobe, whereas craniopharyngioma occurs in the third ventricle. CT scan and particularly MRI are essential in diagnosis. Patchy intracerebral calcification may develop in tuberous sclerosis, an autosomal dominant disease characterized by the triad of epilepsy, mental retardation, and facial skin lesions (multiple angiofibromas). In addition, subependymal gliosis, cardiac rhabdomyoma, renal angiomyolipoma, and periungual fibroma occur. Calcification of the basal ganglia occurs in about 20 percent of patients with chronic hypoparathyroidism, which sometimes leads to a parkinsonian syndrome.

410. The answer is E. *(Robbins, 4/e. pp 1387–1388.)* The neuroglial cells—astrocytes, oligodendrocytes, ependymal cells, and microglial cells—provide supportive and protective functions for neurons. However, only microglial cells are phagocytic and, in response to injury or destruction of the brain, become activated as macrophages (gitter cells, compound granular corpuscles). Astrocytes support neurons and react to CNS injury by formation of glial scars (gliosis). Oligodendrocytes produce and maintain CNS myelin, and diseases affecting them include multiple sclerosis and the leukodystrophies. The lining ependymal cells do not produce or absorb cerebrospinal fluid. Cell processes of astrocytes, or "glial" fibers, contain vimentin and glial fibrillary acidic protein (GFAP).

411. The answer is D. *(Robbins, 4/e. pp 1389–1390, 1409–1411.)* The clinical constellation of altered sensorium and papilledema should call to mind the presence of intracranial pressure, regardless of the cause, which can be due to cerebral edema, tumor mass, or, more commonly, intracranial bleeding with hematoma formation. If the pressure is severe enough, downward displacement of the cerebellar tonsils into the foramen magnum may occur, producing further compression on the brainstem with consequent hemorrhage into the pons and midbrain (Duret hemorrhages). This is nearly always associated with death, since the vital centers, including respiratory control, are located in these regions. Subdural as well as epidural hemorrhages are sufficient to cause critical downward displacement of the cerebellar tonsils. The situation can be remedied with appropriate neurosurgical intervention. In this situation, the downward displacement could be due to hemorrhage-hematoma formation into the posterior intracranial fossa, caused by either a direct (coup) or an indirect (contracoup) blow to the occiput.

412. The answer is C. *(Fitzpatrick, 2/e. pp 584–587. Robbins, 4/e. pp 139–140.)* In von Hippel–Lindau disease, a rare autosomal dominant disorder, multiple benign and malignant neoplasms occur. These include hemangioblastomas of retina and brain (cerebellum and medulla oblongata), angiomas of kidney and liver, and renal cell carcinoma in 25 to 50 percent of cases. Classic neurofibromatosis (NF-1) is characterized by café-au-lait skin macules, axillary freckling, multiple neurofibromas, and Lisch nodules (pigmented iris hamartomas). Lisch nodules are found in 95 percent of patients after age 6, and axillary freckles are almost pathognomonic for the disease. Hamartomas of the iris are not present in central or acoustic neurofibromatosis (NF-2), and though both types of neurofibromatosis have café-au-lait macules and neurofibromas, only the central, or acoustic, form has bilateral acoustic neuromas. The classic form may have unilateral acoustic neuroma. There is increased risk of developing meningiomas or even pheochromocytoma. The gene for the classic form is located on chromosome 17 and the gene encoding the nerve growth factor receptor has been mapped to the same region of chromosome 17.

413. The answer is B. *(Robbins, 4/e. pp 1432–1433.)* ALS, which is a disease of unknown cause with no effective treatment, is fatal in 2 to 6 years. It results in progressive loss of upper and lower motor neuron function. Early symptoms include limb weakness and cramping, then muscle atrophy and fasciculations, often in the hands and arms, but also in a leg (loss of lower motor neurons). Reflexes are hyperactive in upper and lower extremities, and a positive extensor plantar (Babinski) reflex occurs (loss of upper motor neurons). Early in the disease, upper motor neuron signs may predominate, with resultant spasticity of some muscles. The triad of atrophic weakness of hands and forearms, slight spasticity of the legs, and generalized hyperreflexia—in the absence of sensory changes—suggests the diagnosis. There is atrophy and loss of cells in the anterior gray horns and of motor nuclei of the lower brainstem, with bilateral degeneration of the pyramidal tracts that results in mixed upper and lower motor neuron disease. Symptoms of brainstem involvement include dysarthria and dysphagia. Variants of motor neuron disease include progressive muscular atrophy with only lower motor neuron signs and primary lateral sclerosis with only upper motor neuron signs and symptoms.

414. The answer is E. *(Robbins, 4/e. pp 1272–1273.)* Primary tumors of the pineal gland are very uncommon but are of interest, especially in view of the mysterious and relatively unknown functions of the pineal gland itself. The gland secretes neurotransmitter substances such as serotonin and dopamine, with the major product being melatonin. Tumors of the pineal gland include germ cell tumors of all types including embryonal carcinoma, choriocarcinoma, teratoma, and various combinations of germinomas. Germ cell tumors may arise extragonadally within the retroperitoneal space and the pineal gland, with the only commonality being that these structures are in the midline. Primary tumors of the pineal gland occur in two forms: the pineoblastoma and the pineocytoma. Pineoblastomas occur in young patients and consist of small tumors having areas of hemorrhage and necrosis with pleomorphic nuclei and frequent mitoses. Pineocytomas occur in older adults and are slow-growing; they are better differentiated and have large rosettes. Craniopharyngiomas occur not in the pineal gland but above the pituitary gland in the hypothalamus and are thought to arise from structures related to Rathke's pouch.

415. The answer is A. *(Robbins, 4/e. pp 963–964, 1399–1402.)* Subacute sclerosing panencephalitis (SSPE) is caused by the measles virus following infection early in life. There is a long latent period, protracted course, and high mortality. Histopathologic and electron-microscopic changes include perivascular mononuclear cell infiltrates, extensive neuronal loss, and intranuclear inclusions containing paramyxovirus particles in oligodendrocytes and neurons. The CSF contains oligoclonal immunoglobulins against viral components.

Progressive multifocal leukoencephalopathy (PML) is a viral infection of myelin-producing oligodendrocytes and causes primary demyelination. Oligodendroglial nuclei are enlarged and contain inclusion bodies, and bizarre giant astrocytes and foamy macrophages with myelin debris are seen in lesions. Electron microscopy reveals papovavirus particles in oligodendrocyte nuclei. Reye's syndrome occurs within 3 to 5 days of viral infection (influenza, chickenpox) treated with aspirin and is associated with severe or fatal brain edema. Creutzfeldt-Jakob disease, a spongiform encephalopathy, and kuru are probably transmitted by unconventional agents, or prions, that do not appear to be conventional viruses.

416. The answer is B. *(Robbins, 4/e. p 1441.)* Syringomyelia is a chronic myelopathy. There is cavitation involving the central gray matter of the spinal cord where pain fibers cross to join the contralateral spinothalamic tract. Interruption of the lateral spinothalamic tracts results in segmental sensory dissociation, with loss of pain and temperature sense, but preservation of the sense of touch and pressure, or vibration, usually over the neck, shoulders, and arms. Characteristic features also include wasting of the small intrinsic hand muscles (clawhand) and thoracic scoliosis. The cause of syringomyelia is unknown, although one type is associated with a Chiari malformation with obstruction at the foramen magnum.

417. The answer is D. *(Robbins, 4/e. pp 684, 1834.)* Chronic deficiency of cobalamin (vitamin B_{12}) has two major effects: a macrocytic megaloblastic anemia and a spinal cord degeneration, which may precede the anemia by months. The posterior columns and lateral corticospinal tracts undergo myelin degeneration, but the gray matter is rarely affected. Motor weakness with spasticity is the characteristic result, preceded by persistent paresthesias of the feet and hands. SCD is due to failure of the cobalamin-dependent enzyme methylmalonic CoA mutase, which is essential for maintenance of myelinated fibers. The classic triad of dermatitis, diarrhea, and dementia occurs in pellagra, which is due to niacin/nicotinic acid (Vitamin B_5) deficiency.

418. The answer is D. *(Robbins, 4/e. p 1394.)* Tabes dorsalis causes bilateral degeneration of dorsal nerve roots and the posterior funiculi. During the early phase of the disease, there are sharp attacks of pain because of irritation of the dorsal nerve roots, but later there is a progressive loss of sensitivity to pain, vibration, and proprioceptive stimuli. Argyll Robertson pupils are observed, and the interruption of the stretch reflex may result in a positive Romberg sign. The pathogenesis of tabes dorsalis is controversial. Etiologic postulates include focal leptomeningeal inflammation of the dorsal roots, such factors as changes in the structure of the dorsal root ganglia, and a toxic product or metabolic disorder rather than tissue infestation by *Treponema*.

419. The answer is C. *(Anderson, 9/e. pp 1082, 1089.)* The photomicrograph (at low magnification) shows an intact overlying mucosa with a subjacent highly cellular neoplasm composed of small, dark-staining cells ("tumor of small blue cells"). In the child, small, blue cell tumors comprise lymphoma, neuroblastoma, cerebellar medulloblastoma, undifferentiated nephroblastoma (Wilms' tumor), retinoblastoma, embryonal rhabdomyosarcoma, and Ewing's sarcoma. In the adult, anaplastic, small cell carcinomas of the lung, pancreas, uterine cervix, and anorectum (cloacogenic carcinoma); plasmacytomas; and neuroectodermal tumors of thoracopulmonary origin are also included. In addition to the age of the patient and the organ site, certain structures visible at higher magnification, such as rosettes (retinoblastoma) and pseudorosettes (anaplastic small cell carcinoma, neuroblastoma) aid in the differential diagnosis. In the example given, the lesion is too cellular to be either nasal glioma (large, pale glial cells) or nasopharyngeal angiofibroma (vascular structures). The olfactory neuroblastoma (the tumor depicted in the photomicrograph) arises from the olfactory placode of the stem cell referred to as the *esthesioneuroblast*. The cells populating the tumor are round or oval neuroepithelial cells occurring in clusters and associated with a fibrillary intercellular matrix.

420. The answer is D. *(Robbins, 4/e. pp 1426–1429.)* Alzheimer's disease (AD) is characterized by numerous neurofibrillary tangles and senile plaques with a central core of amyloid β-protein. Both tangles and plaques are found to a lesser extent in other conditions, e.g., neurofibrillary tangles in Down's syndrome. Silver stains demonstrate tangles and plaques and Congo red shows amyloid deposition in plaques and vascular walls (amyloid angiopathy). In AD there are also numerous Hirano bodies, and granulovacuolar degeneration is found in more than 10 percent of the neurons of the hippocampus. AD often begins insidiously with impairment of memory and progresses to dementia. Grossly, brain atrophy (narrowed gyri and widened sulci) is predominant in frontal and superior temporal lobes. Lewy bodies are found in idiopathic parkinsonism and in diffuse Lewy body disease.

421–425. The answers are: 421-C, 422-A, 423-B, 424-C, 425-D. *(Robbins, 4/e. pp 1438–1439.)* Developmental anomalies of the central nervous system occur under genetic and environmental influences or sporadically during a critical phase in gestation. Various trisomies are examples of genetic mishaps. Environmental factors include drugs (both therapeutic and illegal), ionizing radiation, infections (rubella, syphilis, toxoplasmosis), malnutrition, and circulatory insufficiency.

When the bony spinal cord fails to close, multiple errors, occurring sporadically as single entities or in association with other central nervous system anomalies, are possible. Spina bifida, the most common developmental defect that occurs in the neural tube, involves the failure of the vertebral arches to close completely. Meningomyelocele is herniation of part of the spinal cord tissue and the meninges through such a defect. In spina bifida occulta the defect in the closure of the neural tube is covered by skin and dermis, with only a pinpoint sinus or hair-covered depression marking the site. Bacterial meningitis, or meningomyelitis, is the major potential risk in these patients.

A developmental defect in the skull bones similar to spina bifida is cranium bifidum, which is regarded as a congenital cranial cleft. Meningocele is herniation of the meninges alone through a cranium bifidum.

Meningoencephalocele includes herniation of meninges and brain substance in the region of the occipital bone. Meningoencephalocystocele, a herniation at the roof of the mouth, together with cranial meningocele and cranial meningoencephalocele, occurs less frequently than the herniations associated with spina bifida.

The Arnold-Chiari malformation consists of herniation of the cerebellum and fourth ventricle into the foramen magnum, skull base flattening, and cerebral aqueduct stenosis with hydrocephalus and meningomyelocele. Various combinations of the above abnormalities exist, and it not necessary for all of them to be uniformly present for the disease to qualify as Arnold-Chiari malformation. In all cases, however, the clinical course is reflected by the degree of hydrocephalus.

426–432. The answers are: 426-B, 427-E, 428-C, 429-D, 430-A, 431-D, 432-C. *(Robbins, 4/e. pp 144–147, 1422–1426, 1429–1430, 1436–1438.)* Tay-Sachs disease (GM_2 gangliosidosis type I) is one of the lysosomal storage diseases and, more specifically, is one of the sphingolipidoses. Absence of hexosaminidase A leads to accumulation of ganglioside in neurons of the central and autonomic nervous systems and retina. Neurons appear swollen and vacuolated with lysosomes filled with gangliosides. The characteristic cherry-red spot in the macula (due to contrasting gangliosidic retinal pallor) may also be seen in up to 50 percent of cases of Niemann-Pick disease, in which sphingomyelin accumulates.

Major histologic features of Alzheimer's disease include neurofibrillary tangles, neuritic (senile) plaques, amyloid angiopathy, granulovacuolar degeneration, and Hirano bodies. Genetic studies have revealed a genetic defect on chromosome 21 in familial Alzheimer's disease with the gene that codes for the amyloid protein also on chromosome 21, though not in the exact location of the genetic defect of familial Alzheimer's disease.

In primary CNS demyelination there is loss of myelin sheaths but relative preservation of axons. This type of demyelination is seen predominantly in multiple sclerosis, in the perivenous encephalomyelopathies (acute disseminated encephalomyelitis and acute hemorrhagic leukoencephalitis), and in progressive multifocal leukoencephalopathy. Secondary CNS demyelination occurs because of destruction of the axons themselves.

Multiple sclerosis of unknown etiology causes disseminated but focal plaques of primary demyelination in gray and white matter anywhere in the CNS, but often near the angles of the lateral ventricles. It affects adults between 20 and 40 years of age who may have nystagmus, tremor, dysarthria, paresthesias, and incoordination. A relapsing and remitting course is usual.

In acute disseminated encephalomyelitis (postinfectious or postvaccinial) there are many foci of perivenous demyelination. It occurs, rarely, after a viral infection (measles, mumps, chickenpox) but is not a slow viral infection. Although the disease is fatal in up to 20 percent of cases, prognosis in survivors is quite good.

Abnormal or defective myelin metabolism is characteristic of Krabbe's disease (globoid cell leukodystrophy) and metachromatic leukodystrophy. These leukodystrophies or inborn errors of metabolism usually appear in early childhood. Metachromatic leukodystrophy is an autosomal recessive disorder of sphingomyelin metabolism and results from deficiency of cerebroside sulfatase (aryl-sulfatase A). Sulfatides accumulate in lysosomes and stain metachromatically with cresyl violet. Diagnostic measures include amniocentesis, enzyme analysis, and measuring decreased urinary aryl-sulfatase A. Demyelination is widespread in the cerebrum and peripheral nervous system. Krabbe's disease, also autosomal recessive, is marked by accumulation of galactocerebroside, demyelination, and multinucleate histiocytes (globoid cells) in the white matter.

Huntington's disease is autosomal dominant with its defective gene on chromosome 4. It involves the extrapyramidal system and causes atrophy of the caudate nuclei and putamen. Choreiform movements and progressive dementia seldom appear before age 30.

433–439. The answers are: 433-A, 434-F, 435-B, 436-D, 437-A, 438-E, 439-C. (*Robbins, 4/e. pp 956, 1397, 1425, 1431, 1445–1446.*) In classic, or idiopathic, parkinsonism (Parkinson's disease) there is degeneration and loss of pigmented cells in the substantia nigra. With less than 25 percent of nigral cells remaining, there is a deficiency of dopamine in the nigral cells, where dopamine is synthesized, and at the synaptic endings of nigral fibers in the striatum. The severity of the motor syndrome correlates with the degree of dopamine deficiency. Lewy bodies, eosinophilic intracytoplasmic inclusions, are found in remaining neurons of the substantia nigra and are largely localized there in classic Parkinson's disease, unlike diffuse Lewy body disease.

Postencephalitic parkinsonism (von Economo's disease), one of the complications of encephalitis lethargica, is similar to classic Parkinson's disease in degeneration of the striatonigral pathway with diminished dopamine and depigmentation in the corpus striatum. However, it occurs earlier and is not progressive. In postencephalitic parkinsonism, neurofibrillary tangles, which are thickened and tortuous neurofilaments stainable by silver, form within neurons.

In Pick's disease, a presenile dementia, neurofibrillary tangles are also demonstrable, but they are fewer than in either Alzheimer's disease or postencephalitic parkinsonism. Pick's disease is a major cortical degenerative disease associated with marked atrophy of frontal lobes and partial temporal lobe atrophy.

Herpes simplex encephalitis presents a high mortality if not treated with vidarabine (adenine arabinoside, ara-A). It causes necrotizing lesions with Cowdry A intranuclear inclusions in oligodendroglia and occasional neurons. Perivascular mononuclear infiltrates occur and hemorrhagic necrosis is present in the temporal and frontal lobes, especially the orbital gyri.

Wilson's disease (hepatolenticular degeneration) is inherited as a primary defect in copper metabolism with increased copper in liver (cirrhosis) and brain (cavitation). Degenerative cavitation or brown discoloration occurs mainly in the lenticular nucleus and thalamus, and copper pigmentation in the cornea (Kayser-Fleischer rings) is distinctive.

Schwannomas (neurilemmomas) are single, encapsulated tumors of nerve sheaths, usually benign, occurring on peripheral, spinal, or cranial nerves. The acoustic neuroma is one example. Microscopically, Verocay bodies, which are foci of palisaded nuclei, may be found in the more cellular (Antoni A) tissue.

Devic's syndrome (neuromyelitis optica) is a variant of multiple sclerosis with rapid onset of demyelination of the optic nerve and of the spinal cord with paraplegia. A pleocytosis with polymorphonuclear cells and a protein content higher than is usual in multiple sclerosis may be seen in cerebrospinal fluid.

Musculoskeletal System

DIRECTIONS: Each question below contains five suggested responses. Select the **one best** response to each question.

440. The most common tumor that involves bone is

(A) a metastatic tumor from an extraosseous site
(B) osteogenic sarcoma
(C) multiple myeloma
(D) chondrosarcoma
(E) a giant cell tumor

441. Which of the following statements about osteoid osteoma is true?

(A) It occurs predominantly in adults
(B) Pain occurs predominantly at night
(C) It is associated occasionally with Gardner's syndrome
(D) It is frequently located in the spine
(E) Occasional malignant change occurs

442. Tuberculous spondylitis (Pott's disease) is characterized by all the following EXCEPT

(A) involvement of thoracic and lumbar vertebrae
(B) hematogenous spread
(C) proliferative synovitis with pannus
(D) destruction of intervertebral disks
(E) formation of psoas abscess

443. The part of a long bone initially involved in hematogenous osteomyelitis is the

(A) metaphyseal region
(B) diaphysis
(C) epiphysis
(D) area around the entrance of the nutrient artery
(E) medullary cavity

444. All the following statements
about chondrosarcoma are true
EXCEPT that

(A) it is most frequent in middle age
      or later
(B) the peripheral type can arise
      from enchondroma
(C) it is common in the pelvic bones
(D) histologic analysis is of prognos-
      tic significance
(E) it is the second most common
      malignant bone tumor

---

445. All the following diseases may be associated with the grossly deformed joint depicted in the photograph below EXCEPT

(A) leprosy
(B) psoriasis
(C) syringomyelia
(D) pernicious anemia
(E) diabetes mellitus

446. The lesion illustrated in the photomicrograph below is most likely

(A) a rheumatoid nodule
(B) myositis ossificans
(C) necrotizing panniculitis
(D) polymyositis
(E) fat necrosis

447. Bilateral segmental osteone-
crosis or avascular necrosis (AVN)
of the femoral head is most often associated with

(A) systemic steroid therapy
(B) irradiation therapy
(C) sickle cell disease
(D) alcoholism
(E) fracture of the femoral neck

448. Osteogenesis imperfecta type I
is characterized by

(A) a hereditary defect in osteoclas-
     tic function
(B) defective synthesis of type II
     collagen
(C) defective synthesis of osteoid
     matrix
(D) early death
(E) bone marrow aplasia

---

449. The specimen shown in the photomicrograph below is from a mass removed from the thigh of a 58-year-old man. Using the current nomencla-
ture, this lesion is compatible with

(A) nodular fasciitis
(B) rhabdomyosarcoma
(C) myositis ossificans
(D) osteogenic sarcoma
(E) malignant fibrous histiocytoma

450. The bone disease shown below in the photomicrograph of a bone biopsy is associated with all the following EXCEPT

(A) excessive bone resorption
(B) high serum levels of alkaline phosphatase
(C) elevated serum levels of calcium
(D) polyostotic occurrence
(E) pathologic fractures

451. Which of the following fibroosseous bone disorders is most likely to be associated with skin lesions?

(A) Osteoid osteoma
(B) Albright's syndrome
(C) Nonossifying fibroma
(D) Polyostotic fibrous dysplasia
(E) Monostotic fibrous dysplasia

452. A perivascular inflammatory infiltrate in skeletal muscle, as shown in the photomicrograph below, is likely to be seen in all the following EXCEPT

(A) hypersensitivity angiitis
(B) polymyositis
(C) polyarteritis nodosa
(D) cystic medial necrosis
(E) systemic sclerosis

---

453. Giant cell tumors of bone (osteoclastomas) are known to have all the following characteristics EXCEPT

(A) they occur rarely under the age of 15
(B) they occur commonly around the knee
(C) they show unpredictable biologic behavior
(D) they arise in the epiphyseal ends of long bones
(E) they have a recurrence rate of 10 percent

454. The atypical rhabdomyoblasts illustrated in the photomicrograph below may be seen in all the following lesions EXCEPT

(A) sarcoma botryoides
(B) myositis ossificans
(C) mixed heterologous müllerian tumor of the uterus
(D) adult pleomorphic rhabdomyosarcoma
(E) embryonal rhabdomyosarcoma

---

455. A sex-linked recessive mode of inheritance exists in

(A) myotonic dystrophy
(B) limb-girdle dystrophy
(C) facioscapulohumeral dystrophy
(D) Duchenne's muscular dystrophy
(E) polymyositis

456. True statements about the tumor shown below in a radiograph of a
hemisected tibia include all the following EXCEPT

(A) it constitutes about 20 percent of all primary malignant bone tumors
(B) it may have a sunburst appearance on x-ray
(C) it is a juxtacortical (parosteal) osteosarcoma
(D) it has a 5-year survival rate of 60 percent with combined therapy
(E) it may be associated with Paget's disease in the elderly

457. In the disorder depicted below in which multiple, focal osteolytic skull lesions occur, all the following are common EXCEPT

(A) a normal serum alkaline phosphatase level
(B) increased production of monoclonal immunoglobulin
(C) lymphadenopathy
(D) bone pain
(E) hypercalcemia

DIRECTIONS: Each group of questions below consists of lettered headings followed by a set of numbered items. For each numbered item select the **one** lettered heading with which it is **most** closely associated. Each lettered heading may be used **once, more than once, or not at all.**

Questions 458–462

For each disease choose the artist's representation of a microradiogram, shown below, with which it is most likely to be associated. Answer "E" if the disease is not associated with any of the microradiograms.

E None of the above

458. Primary hyperparathyroidism

459. Vitamin D–resistant rickets

460. Osteoporosis

461. Paget's disease

462. Osteopetrosis

Questions 463–466

For each bone lesion, select the lettered location and general configuration with which it is most likely to be associated in the diagram.

463. Giant cell tumor of bone (osteoclastoma)

464. Unicameral (solitary) bone cyst

465. Osteochondroma

466. Nonossifying fibroma of bone

DIRECTIONS: The group of questions below consists of four lettered headings followed by a set of numbered items. For each numbered item select

A	if the item is associated with	(A) **only**
B	if the item is associated with	(B) **only**
C	if the item is associated with	**both** (A) and (B)
D	if the item is associated with	**neither** (A) nor (B)

Each lettered heading may be used **once, more than once, or not at all.**

Questions 467–470

(A) Ewing's sarcoma of bone
(B) Osteogenic sarcoma
(C) Both
(D) Neither

467. Peak incidence at ages 10 to 20

468. Glycogen-positive tumor cells on PAS staining

469. Absence of significant radiographic findings

470. Prior irradiation

Musculoskeletal System
Answers

440. The answer is A. *(Anderson, 9/e. pp 2055–2056.)* Metastases account for the majority of bone tumors, followed in frequency by multiple myeloma and osteogenic sarcoma. Common carcinomas that metastasize to bone include lung, thyroid, breast, prostate, and renal cell carcinomas. Whereas most metastatic carcinomas to bone produce osteolytic radiologic lesions, prostate carcinoma tends to produce osteoblastic metastases. The serum calcium and alkaline phosphatase may be elevated in osseous metastases.

441. The answer is B. *(Bullough, pp 11.13–11.17, 12.2–12.3. Robbins, 4/e. pp 896, 1335–1336.)* Osteoid osteoma (OO) occurs predominantly in children or young adults in the second and third decades of life as a benign osteoblastic (bone-forming) lesion of small size, usually less than 1 cm. In osteoid osteoma malignant change does not occur, unlike the closely related but larger osteoblastoma, in which there is occasional malignant change. OO is often located in the diaphyseal cortex of tibia or femur, unlike osteoblastoma, which occurs in the spine (vertebral arch) or medulla of long bones. Rarely, osteoma, another osteoblastic tumor, is associated with Gardner's syndrome, in which colonic polyposis and osteomas, epidermal cysts, and fibromatosis occur. Night pain, relieved by salicylates, is prominent with OO. OO consists of a very small, often radiolucent nidus of slender, mineralized osteoid trabeculae with intervening connective tissue; the entire lesion is enclosed by dense sclerotic bone. Treatment is complete excision of the nidus to prevent recurrence. Since osteonectin antibodies immunolocalize osteonectin in osteoblasts, these antibodies react with bone-forming tumors, benign or malignant.

442. The answer is C. *(Robbins, 4/e. pp 1322, 1354.)* Pott's disease of the spine is caused by tuberculous infection of the lower thoracic and lumbar vertebrae. Destruction of the intervertebral disks and adjacent vertebral bodies causes them to collapse, and these compression fractures may result in angular kyphosis or scoliosis. Caseous material may extend from the vertebrae into paravertebral muscles and along the psoas muscle sheath to form a psoas abscess in the inguinal regions. Tuberculous osteomyelitis occurs most often in the long bones and spine and via hematogenous spread from a primary site elsewhere. Chronic proliferative synovitis with pannus formation is characteristic of rheumatoid arthritis and Lyme arthritis. In Lyme arthritis there is also hyperplastic "onionskin" arteriolar thickening (similar to that in syphilis).

443. The answer is A. *(Robbins, 4/e. pp 1320–1322.)* Nutrient arteries to long bones divide to supply the metaphyses and diaphyses. In the metaphyses, the arteries become arterioles and finally form capillary loops adjacent to epiphyseal plates. This anatomic feature allows bacteria to settle in the region of the metaphysis and makes it the site initially involved in hematogenous osteomyelitis. As a consequence of vascular and osteoclastic resorption, the infected bone is replaced by fibrous connective tissue. Persistent chronic osteomyelitis is often associated with sequelae that include amyloidosis and the appearance of malignant tumors in old sinus tracts within the damaged bone.

444. The answer is E. *(Robbins, 4/e. pp 1340–1342.)* Chondrosarcoma shows a peak incidence in the sixth and seventh decades. Most chondrosarcomas (85 percent) arise de novo, but the peripheral type, unlike the central type, may arise in benign tumors of cartilage, especially if they are multiple. Frequent sites of origin include pelvic bones (50 percent), humerus, femur, ribs, and spine. Although a fairly common form of bone cancer, chondrosarcoma is preceded in frequency by metastatic carcinoma, multiple myeloma, and osteosarcoma. Histologic grading is most important in prognosis since grade I and grade II lesions present very good 5-year survival rates following surgery, unlike grade III, poorly differentiated tumors, which invade quickly and metastasize to lungs.

445. The answer is B. *(Anderson, 9/e. pp 2068, 2158. Bullough, p 7.16.)* The photograph displays a grossly deformed knee joint, an example of neurogenic arthropathy (Charcot's joint). This is a rapidly destructive, often monarticular form of osteoarthritis. Destruction of the joint surface, subluxation or dislocation, and loose bodies are prominent, and the scarred, chronically inflamed synovium contains striking bone and cartilage detritus. The underlying neurologic lesion with its resultant loss of local proprioception and sensory nerve paths may occur in tabes dorsalis, syringomyelia, leprosy, diabetes, spina bifida, or chronic alcoholism. The rare association of arthritis and psoriasis characteristically affects the distal interphalangeal joints of hands and feet in asymmetric fashion.

446. The answer is A. *(Anderson, 9/e. pp 2079, 2082–2083.)* Rheumatoid arthritis frequently affects the small joints of the hands and feet. The larger joints are involved later. Subcutaneous nodules, with a necrotic focus surrounded by palisades of proliferating cells, are seen in some cases. In the joints, the synovial membrane is thickened by a granulation tissue pannus that is infiltrated by many inflammatory cells. Nodular collections of lymphocytes resembling follicles are characteristically seen. The thickened synovial membrane may develop villous projections, and the joint cartilage is attacked and destroyed.

447. The answer is A. *(Anderson, 9/e. pp 163–164. Bullough, pp 7.2–7.8.)* AVN of bone is a moderately frequent complication of high-dose systemic corticosteroid therapy—the usual cause of bilateral segmental infarction or AVN of the femoral head. Clinical features include sudden onset of severe pain and difficulty in walking, with AVN accounting for about 20 percent of hip diseases that require prosthetic replacement. Within the femoral head a triangular yellow area of necrotic bone is found beneath the viable articular cartilage, and x-ray may show a crescent sign or space between cartilage and underlying infarct. Fracture of the subcapital femoral neck is frequently associated with unilateral AVN; the other conditions listed are much less frequently associated.

448. The answer is C. *(Bullough, pp 3.2–3.8. Robbins, 4/e. p 1318.)* Osteogenesis imperfecta (OI), or brittle bone disease, constitutes a group of disorders often inherited as autosomal dominant traits and caused by genetic mutations involving the synthesis of type I collagen, which comprises about 90 percent of the osteoid, or bone matrix. Very early perinatal death and multiple fractures occur in OI type II, which is often autosomal recessive. The major variant of OI, type I, is compatible with survival; after the perinatal period fractures occur in addition to other signs of defective collagen synthesis such as thin, translucent, blue sclerae; laxity of joint ligaments; deafness from otosclerosis; and abnormal teeth. A hereditary defect in osteoclastic function with decreased bone resorption and bone overgrowth, which sometimes narrows or obliterates the marrow cavity, is characteristic of osteopetrosis, or marble bone disease.

449. The answer is E. *(Anderson, 9/e. pp 1853–1860.)* Malignant fibrous histiocytoma (MFH) is the current term used to designate sarcomatous growths of the deep soft tissues. This is principally a disease of the lower extremity and thigh in middle- to advanced-aged patients of both sexes, but it has also been reported as occurring in far-removed areas, such as the adventitia of the thoracic aorta and the ocular orbit. It has also occurred with some frequency years after irradiation. The tumor is composed of a background of spindle cells with varying amounts of collagen (hence, fibrous) and scattered, giant, bizarre, xanthomatous and myoblastic-like cells (hence, histiocytic). In the past, many of these tumors were undoubtedly labeled as "pleomorphic liposarcomas" and "pleomorphic adult rhabdomyosarcomas," both of which must be differentiated from MFH. This does not imply, of course, that pleomorphic liposarcomas and adult rhabdomyosarcomas do not exist simply because a new term has been introduced, but rather that strict histologic criteria should be adhered to in order to exclude MFH—namely, that malignant myoblasts with cytoplasmic striations (rhabdomyosarcoma) and lipoblasts (liposarcoma) must be unequivocally demonstrated. The prognosis is poor for MFH.

450. The answer is C. *(Anderson, 9/e. pp 2006–2011.)* Paget's disease, or osteitis deformans, is characterized by excessive resorption of bone and replacement by abnormally soft, poorly mineralized matrix. Since formation of new bone occurs almost simultaneously, serum levels of calcium are normal. Serum levels of alkaline phosphatase are usually higher than in any other bone disorder. Pathologic fractures are fairly frequent in vertebrae (back pain), tibia, femur, or humerus. Polyostotic occurrence is more usual than monostotic. Histologically, the mosaic pattern of cement lines traversing thick, irregular bone trabeculae is characteristic of the sclerotic, or late, phase of Paget's disease (abnormally hard bone).

451. The answer is B. *(Robbins, 4/e. pp 1331–1336.)* Fibroosseous lesions of bone classically include fibrous dysplasia (FD), nonossifying fibroma (fibrous cortical defect), and osteoid osteoma. Histologically, FD shows a characteristic "Chinese-lettering" effect of the bony trabeculae, which are surrounded by a cellular, fibrous stroma, with osteoblasts and osteoclasts conspicuously decreased at the periphery of the entrapped woven bone. Histologically, nonossifying fibroma shows characteristic foam cell histiocytes within the lesions of the metaphysis. Osteoid osteomas are found within the diaphysis of long bones and contain osteoid trabeculae in a cellular, fibrous matrix, but unlike FD, this disease demonstrates (singular) peripheral trabecular osteoblasts. FD produces radiolucent bone lesions involving long bones and thorax, skull, and facial bones. *Monostotic FD* refers to single-bone involvement, *polyostotic FD* refers to involvement of multiple lesions or bones, and *Albright's syndrome* refers to polyostotic bone lesions, endocrinopathy (hyperthyroidism, thyrotoxicosis, hyperpituitarism, Cushing's syndrome), precocious puberty in females, and café-au-lait spots on the skin. The pigmented, macular café-au-lait spots are usually more irregular ("coast of Maine") in outline than the forms seen in neurofibromatosis. Monostotic FD is very rarely associated with the skin lesions.

452. The answer is D. *(Robbins, 4/e. pp 138, 208–210, 571–574.)* Cystic medial necrosis is not inflammatory, but degenerative. Hypersensitivity angiitis primarily affects small vessels; polyarteritis nodosa affects small to medium-sized arteries. In addition to interstitial inflammation (often perivascular), patients with polymyositis have histologic evidence of muscle fiber death. Perivascular inflammation is one of the early skeletal muscle changes in scleroderma (systemic sclerosis).

453. The answer is E. *(Anderson, 9/e. pp 2043–2045.)* Giant cell tumors of bone arise eccentrically in long-bone epiphyses, most commonly around the knee, in young to middle-aged adults (20 to 55 years) and are rare under 15 years of age. They show unpredictable and variable biologic behavior; even lesions that appear benign may recur following therapy, the overall recurrence rate being 25 to 50 percent. The fibroblast-like, prominent, spindle cell tumor stroma forms the neoplastic element, and the numerous giant cells with features of osteoclasts, scattered regularly throughout the lesion, do not. Many lesions with numerous giant cells simulate it, but it has definite characteristics—it is grossly hemorrhagic, reddish-brown, and gray with central cystic degeneration and a fairly typical x-ray appearance of a lobulated, lytic lesion within the epiphysis.

454. The answer is B. *(Robbins, 4/e. pp 1373–1377, 1381–1382.)* Myositis ossificans is a benign condition characterized by fibrous repair of a skeletal muscle or subcutaneous fat, hematoma with secondary cartilage formation, ossification, and calcification. The other lesions mentioned are malignant neoplasms that may contain a variety of mesodermal tissues. Many tumors diagnosed as rhabdomyosarcoma in the past would be classified as malignant fibrous histiocytoma today, although if cell striations are present in the cells, the lesions still qualify as rhabdomyosarcoma.

455. The answer is D. *(Anderson, 9/e. pp 2111–2112.)* Classification of the muscular dystrophies is based on the mode of inheritance and clinical features. Inheritance of the Duchenne type is by an X-linked recessive trait, with the gene located on the short arm of the X chromosome, although spontaneous mutations are fairly common. Autosomal dominant inheritance characterizes both myotonic dystrophy and the facioscapulohumeral type, while limb-girdle dystrophy is autosomal recessive. In Duchenne's muscular dystrophy, males are affected and symptoms begin before the age of 4. Pelvic-girdle muscles are affected with resultant difficulty in walking, and this is followed by shoulder-girdle weakness and eventual involvement of respiratory and cardiac muscles with death from respiratory failure before age 20. Histologic changes include rounded, atrophic fibers, hypertrophied fibers, degenerative and regenerative changes in adjacent myocytes, and necrotic fibers invaded by histiocytes. Elevation of serum creatine kinase is marked.

456. The answer is C. *(Bullough, pp 12.4–12.12. Robbins, 4/e. pp 1336–1339.)* Juxtacortical (parosteal) osteosarcoma, an uncommon variant of osteogenic sarcoma, is usually a low-grade, slow-growing tumor occurring on an external bone surface. It is found mostly on the posterior lower end of the femur in patients over 20 years of age. Many such tumors have a well-differentiated fibrosarcomatous stroma and, usually, a much better prognosis than does intramedullary osteosarcoma. This tumor may extend through the cortex into the medulla, and CT scan must exclude this before surgical removal, or recurrence may follow. Osteosarcoma is the most common primary malignant bone tumor after multiple myeloma and is the most common bone cancer of children. The characteristic sunburst shown in the x-ray is due to calcified perpendicular striae of reactive periosteum adjacent to the tumor. With surgery, radiation, and chemotherapy the 5-year survival is now about 60 percent. Sometimes DNA analysis is useful in the differential diagnosis of osteosarcoma, since diploid DNA content is usual in benign bone tumors and low-grade parosteal osteosarcoma, while most high-grade osteosarcomas are hyperploid.

457. The answer is C. *(Robbins, 4/e. pp 739–743.)* Multiple myeloma has a peak incidence at 50 to 60 years of age and presents a classic triad of marrow plasmacytosis; a serum or urine M (monoclonal) protein or both, which represent the immunoglobulin molecule (or heavy or light chain) produced by the tumor cells; and lytic bone lesions. Myeloma is a monoclonal malignancy of the B-lymphocyte system with bone pain the most common symptom, and osteolytic, punched-out bone lesions are characteristic, especially in the skull. Since the process is lytic, alkaline phosphatase is usually not raised. Lymphadenopathy occurs in Waldenström's macroglobulinemia, another malignancy of lymphoplasmacytoid cells, but myeloma is not associated with lymphadenopathy. Hypercalcemia from bone resorption is frequent, as are recurrent infections because of severe suppression of normal immunoglobulins. In about 55 percent of patients, the abnormal M component is IgG and in 25 percent it is IgA.

458–462. The answers are: 458-C, 459-D, 460-A, 461-B, 462-E. *(Anderson, 9/e. pp 1949–1952, 1975–1977, 1983–1984, 1993, 2006.)* Primary hyperparathyroidism causes increased size of lacunae in the trabeculae of the bones and is associated with increased levels of parathyroid hormones. Its early lesions consist of loss of calcium and demineralization. For this reason, primary hyperparathyroidism is almost indistinguishable in the early stages from osteomalacia. Osteitis fibrous cystica and "brown tumors" resulting from hyperparathyroidism are very rarely seen today.

Osteoporosis (essential bone loss) causes enlargement of the spaces of bone (the haversian canals) and thus produces a porous appearance in the bones. The loss of bony substance produces a brittleness or softness in the bones. The disease results from either an increased rate of resorption or a decreased rate of bone formation. Osteoporosis can be a manifestation of aging or can be a peripheral effect in a great variety of disorders and other circumstances. These include postmenopause, diabetes mellitus, malnutrition, malabsorption (protein, calcium, vitamin C, and vitamin D deficiencies), Ehlers-Danlos syndrome, Marfan's syndrome, alcohol abuse, heparin administration, methotrexate administration, immobility (such as confinement in bed), and acidosis.

Osteomalacia is demineralization of the osteoid matrix, which results in areas of decreased mineral density and loss of bone rigidity. Rickets is osteomalacia in infants and children. It is usually caused by dietary lack of vitamin D. Osteomalacia in adults is, as it were, vitamin D–resistant rickets. The defect in vitamin D resistance involves a failure of D to be converted to 1,25-$(OH)_2D_3$, which is the metabolically active form of the vitamin. Other examples of this defect are advanced renal disease, or renal osteodystrophy, and congenital absence of 25-hydroxylase.

Paget's disease of bone, or osteitis deformans, is seen late in life. It is a benign disorder of bone characterized by increased skeletal remodeling. The skeletal remodeling is indicated by marked increases both in the amount of resorption activity and in the amount of bone-formation activity. Specifically, there is progressive erosion of cancellous bone spicules, with fibroconnective tissue replacement and eventual concomitant osteoclastic bone resorption with osteoblastic bone formation. A mosaic pattern, caused by persistence of visible osteoid seams, is seen in biopsy material.

Osteopetrosis is a rare hereditary disorder with increased bone mass and density of skeleton and is caused by osteoclast dysfunction (lack of ruffled borders), so that there is reduced bone resorption and bone overgrowth. Loss of the medullary cavity often results in anemia and multiple fractures are frequent. The severe autosomal recessive form causes death in infancy, but the more common autosomal dominant adult form is relatively benign. Osteopetrosis is also known as *marble bone disease.*

463–466. The answers are: 463-A, 464-B, 465-E, 466-D. (*Anderson, 9/e. pp 2021–2022, 2043–2045.*) Osteoclastoma, the giant cell tumor of bone, usually produces a lytic lesion involving the epiphysis of long bones. The proximal tibia is a common site. There are many pitfalls involved in making a diagnosis of giant cell tumor of bone. The main problem involves the difficulty of distinguishing the bone destruction that is a true neoplasm from bone destruction that is the result of various types of osteoclastic-osteoblastic activity. Direct communication with the radiologist and, preferably, the orthopedic surgeon is, therefore, nearly mandatory for the pathologist when making a diagnosis.

Unicameral, or solitary, cysts are loculated, lytic lesions of bone that characteristically abut on the epiphyseal plate in older children and produce cortical irregularities. Regions involved in the benign lesion are prone to fracture.

Osteochondromas are cauliflower-like lesions that contain a core of cortical and medullary bone and a cartilage cap that decreases in width as age increases. They usually protrude from the metaphyses of long bones and may be multiple.

Nonossifying fibromas of bone—usually well-demarcated, eccentric, lytic metaphyseal lesions—most commonly occur in the tibia and femur. They are histologically identical to fibrous cortical defects and consist of a fibroblastic growth without concomitant bone formation.

467–470. The answers are: 467-C, 468-A, 469-D, 470-B. *(Robbins, 4/e. pp 1336–1339, 1342–1343.)* Both Ewing's and osteogenic sarcomas are primary malignant bone tumors that occur predominantly in children and young adults in the second decade of life. However, osteosarcoma can occur in adults over age 40 who have multifocal Paget's disease, or who have been exposed to bone irradiation or to radium-containing paints. Ewing's sarcoma may occur under the age of 10, but is rare under 3. Ewing's tumor usually exhibits glycogen-positive, diastase-sensitive cytoplasmic granules with PAS staining, and electron microscopy demonstrates glycogen in the tumor cells, which is helpful in differentiation from lymphoma and neuroblastoma. Radiographs in osteosarcoma may show periosteal elevation at an acute angle (Codman's triangle) or tumor penetration of cortical bone with extension into the soft tissues. In Ewing's sarcoma reactive new bone formation, subperiosteal and sequential, may cause concentric "onionskin" layering in half the cases. Osteosarcomas usually arise in the metaphyses of long bones of the extremities (lower end of femur, upper end of tibia, upper end of humerus, and upper femur), although they may involve any bone. The origin of Ewing's sarcoma is often the medullary cavity of long bones, innominate bone, or scapula, but the origin may be any bone in diaphysis or metaphysis.

Prognoses for both osteosarcoma and Ewing's tumor have improved in recent years with the combination of surgery and chemotherapy: a 3-year survival of approximately 70 percent in osteogenic sarcoma of osteoblastic type, and a 5-year survival of nearly 70 percent in Ewing's sarcoma. The telangiectatic and the chondroblastic osteosarcomas do not respond as well. Osteosarcomas show marked variation histologically. The malignant osteoblasts may be small and fairly uniform or highly pleomorphic with bizarre shapes and numerous mitoses. If predominantly composed of small, round cells with little tumor osteoid or bone, they can be confused with Ewing's sarcoma.

Skin and Breast

DIRECTIONS: Each question below contains five suggested responses. Select the **one best** response to each question.

471. A menopausal woman is given a diagnosis of lobular carcinoma of the breast. What impact will this have on her clinical follow-up?

(A) The same impact as other types of carcinoma
(B) The impact depends on node involvement
(C) Biopsies of the contralateral breast are indicated
(D) Radiation should be administered
(E) A tylectomy (lumpectomy) is sufficient treatment

472. Mycosis fungoides is correctly characterized by which of the following statements?

(A) It is more common in females
(B) It represents cutaneous spread of a primary nodal lymphoma
(C) It is characterized histologically by microabscesses of Munro
(D) It is a cutaneous lymphoma of T4 cell lineage
(E) It is a cutaneous lymphoma of T8 cell lineage

473. All the following lesions are extremely difficult to differentiate from malignant melanoma on clinical examination alone EXCEPT

(A) seborrheic keratosis
(B) deep penetrating nevus (DPN)
(C) pigmented basal cell carcinoma
(D) thrombosed hemangioma
(E) tufted angioma (angioblastoma)

474. True statements concerning tamoxifen therapy include all the following EXCEPT that

(A) it is the endocrine therapy of choice for advanced breast cancer
(B) it is used for node-negative patients with estrogen-receptor–negative disease
(C) adjuvant tamoxifen therapy is used for all node-negative women with estrogen-receptor–positive disease
(D) adjuvant tamoxifen therapy is used for postmenopausal women with node-positive disease
(E) tamoxifen is under investigation as preventive therapy for healthy women

475. The clinical photograph below suggests that the patient

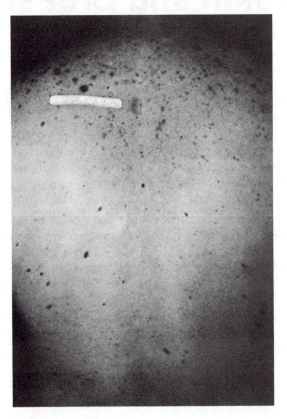

(A) has Leser-Trelat sign
(B) has multiple basal cell nevus syndrome
(C) is at risk for developing malignant melanoma
(D) has leopard syndrome
(E) has Torres's syndrome

476. All the following factors have shown an association with gynecomastia EXCEPT

(A) Leydig cell tumors
(B) seminomas
(C) Sertoli cell tumors
(D) alcoholic cirrhosis
(E) digitalis therapy

477. Malignant or premalignant lesions include all the following EXCEPT

(A) erythroplasia of Queyrat
(B) senile (actinic) keratosis
(C) keratoacanthoma
(D) Bowen's disease
(E) active junctional nevus

478. A number of malignant tumors of the breast have been known in some instances to have a deceptively bland histologic appearance and hence have at times been misdiagnosed as benign by the pathologist. These potentially deceptive tumors include all the following EXCEPT

(A) duct carcinoma
(B) tubular carcinoma
(C) angiosarcoma
(D) papillary carcinoma
(E) metastasizing mucinous carcinoma

479. The most important factor related to the prognosis of breast cancer is

(A) the presence of activated oncogenes
(B) the histologic type and grade
(C) the size of the tumor
(D) the status of axillary lymph nodes
(E) the presence of estrogen receptors

---

480. An excisional biopsy of the nipple area, taken from a 46-year-old woman, is shown below. The patient complained of discharge from the nipple for approximately 4 months. The most likely diagnosis is

(A) fibroadenoma
(B) epidermoid carcinoma
(C) eczematous inflammation
(D) Paget's disease of the breast
(E) mammary fibromatosis

481. The incidence of malignant melanoma of the skin appears to be increasing in the United States. Which of the following is most significant in predicting the clinical behavior following diagnosis?

(A) The degree of pigmentation
(B) The level and depth
(C) The amount of inflammation
(D) The degree of pleomorphism
(E) The state of nutrition

482. Which of the following statements most accurately describes inflammatory breast cancer?

(A) Inflammation improves the prognosis
(B) Inflammation is increased in Paget's disease
(C) Acute inflammatory cells are present
(D) Chronic inflammatory cells are present
(E) Lymphatic permeation is present

483. Which of the following pairs of disorders would most appropriately be considered in the differential diagnosis for the lesion seen in the photomicrograph below?

(A) Superficial spreading malignant melanoma in situ and Paget's disease
(B) Mycosis fungoides and metastatic carcinoma
(C) Psoriasis and lichen planus
(D) Lupus erythematosus and lupus vulgaris
(E) Leukemia and lymphoma

484. A 37-year-old woman presents with a lump in the upper outer quadrant of the left breast, which shows a wide spectrum of benign breast disease on pathologic examination. Which of the following is considered to indicate the greatest risk for subsequent carcinoma of the breast?

(A) Intraductal papillomatosis
(B) Sclerosing adenosis
(C) Florid papillomatosis
(D) Marked apocrine metaplasia
(E) Epithelial hyperplasia of the ducts

485. An adult patient develops crops of bullae and vesicles in the mouth and later on the skin of the trunk. A skin biopsy is inconclusive but shows a suprabasal acantholysis of the overlying epidermis. Direct immunofluorescence of the skin can be used to identify all the following EXCEPT

(A) bullous pemphigoid
(B) pemphigus vulgaris
(C) dermatitis herpetiformis
(D) erythema multiforme
(E) discoid lupus erythematosus (DLE)

486. A 16-year-old girl undergoes biopsy of a breast lump that shows the changes in the photomicrograph below. What is the most appropriate course of action?

(A) Radiotherapy
(B) Local excision
(C) Radical mastectomy
(D) Modified radical mastectomy
(E) No further therapy

487. True statements about the condition seen in the photomicrograph below include all the following EXCEPT

(A) it is often misdiagnosed clinically as seborrheic dermatitis
(B) it may have associated otitis media
(C) it may involve multiple viscera
(D) diabetes mellitus is fairly commonly associated
(E) Birbeck granules can be observed in the cells

488. A papillary lesion is seen in a biopsy from a 32-year-old woman who presented with sanguineous discharge from the nipple. All the following would be useful in differentiating benign intraductal papilloma from papillary adenocarcinoma EXCEPT

(A) a cribriform pattern
(B) knowledge of the presence or absence of cell uniformity
(C) fibrovascular cores
(D) the age of the patient
(E) two cell types (epithelial and myoepithelial)

489. The differential diagnosis of the lesion with dense lymphocytic infiltration depicted below could include all the following EXCEPT

(A) lupus erythematosus
(B) urticaria pigmentosa
(C) polymorphous light eruption
(D) pseudolymphoma
(E) malignant lymphoma

DIRECTIONS: Each group of questions below consists of lettered headings followed by a set of numbered items. For each numbered item select the **one** lettered heading with which it is **most** closely associated. Each lettered heading may be used **once, more than once, or not at all.**

Questions 490–494

Match the characteristic features with the appropriate acanthotic skin disease.

(A) Psoriasis
(B) Lichen planus
(C) Verruca vulgaris
(D) Pemphigus vulgaris
(E) Acanthosis nigricans

490. Elongated, saw-toothed rete ridges and liquefaction degeneration of basal layer

491. Hyperkeratosis, parakeratosis, and vacuolization of the granular layer

492. Papillary, folded hyperkeratosis and melanin pigmentation of basal layer

493. Parakeratosis and elongation of clubbed rete ridges and dermal papillae

494. Microabscesses in the stratum corneum

Questions 495–497

Match each breast disease with the appropriate description.

(A) Is characteristically painful
(B) May present osteoid or chondroid stromal foci
(C) Is frequently bilateral
(D) Never predisposes to carcinoma
(E) Produces scirrhous tumors

495. Ductal carcinoma

496. Sclerosing adenosis

497. Cystosarcoma phyllodes

DIRECTIONS: The group of questions below consists of four lettered headings followed by a set of numbered items. For each numbered item select

A	if the item is associated with	(A) **only**
B	if the item is associated with	(B) **only**
C	if the item is associated with	**both** (A) and (B)
D	if the item is associated with	**neither** (A) nor (B)

Each lettered heading may be used **once, more than once, or not at all.**

Questions 498–500

(A) Marasmus
(B) Kwashiorkor
(C) Both
(D) Neither

498. Thymic atrophy

499. Dermatoses

500. Inelastic wrinkled skin

Skin and Breast
Answers

471. The answer is C. *(Robbins, 4/e. pp 1195, 1198–1199.)* Lobular carcinoma composes up to 10 percent of all histologic types of breast cancer, with duct carcinoma being the most common (70 to 75 percent of the total). It presumably arises from the terminal duct epithelium of the lobule, and it carries a high propensity to multifocality and bilateral breast involvement. There is evidence that this form of breast cancer gives rise to multiple, separate primaries within both breasts. For this reason, breast therapists currently advocate biopsies of the contralateral breast when the tumor is diagnosed. The lobular architectural spectrum begins with lobular hyperplasia and may then progress to lobular neoplasia, atypical lobular neoplasia (lobular carcinoma in situ), and, finally, infiltrating lobular carcinoma. The therapy for lobular hyperplasia and even atypical lobular neoplasia is controversial and is different in various medical centers. If there is any degree of stromal infiltration, however, therapy should at least include a mastectomy; if this is not done, a modified radical mastectomy is required, since the clinical behaviors of infiltrating breast cancers of various histologic subtypes are similar. Some states have written legislation concerning the patient's option to have only excision of the tumor (tylectomy) without mastectomy, since more aggressive conventional surgical therapy has not significantly altered total survival over the past 5 or 6 decades. This new approach should be regarded as controversial, however, and more study is needed before the superiority of alternative forms of therapy over more radical surgery is proved. Early diagnosis still remains the best approach to cancer therapy.

472. The answer is D. *(Robbins, 4/e. pp 1293–1294.)* Mycosis fungoides is part of the spectrum of malignant T-cell lymphomas, mostly of the T4 subset, with a predilection for the skin. It is more common in males and the incidence increases with age. It arises primarily in the skin but more than 70 percent of patients have extracutaneous spread with lymph nodes, spleen, liver, and lungs most often involved. Clinically it presents as cutaneous patches, plaques, or nodules and is often misdiagnosed as psoriasis or other dermatitides. Histologically there is a bandlike infiltrate in the upper dermis of atypical lymphocytes with markedly convoluted nuclei—the Sézary-Lutzner cells. These show epidermotropism and form characteristic intraepidermal clusters known as *Pautrier's microabscesses*. In some cases there is generalized erythroderma and Sézary-Lutzner cells in the peripheral blood. This is known as the Sézary syndrome.

473. The answer is E. *(Fitzpatrick, 2/e. pp 278–283, 330–331, 345, 349–353.)* It is of paramount importance *not* to consider any pigmented skin lesion as benign without adequate excisional biopsy and histologic examination. The first four listed lesions have all caused fairly frequent misdiagnoses, and malignant melanoma has been missed in its early, still curable stage. Seborrheic keratosis is a common, hereditary, benign tumor, usually pigmented and occurring on the trunk, face, and upper extremities after age 30. The mature lesion appears as a plaque with warty, keratotic surface, "stuck on" skin appearance, and horn cysts seen on the surface by hand lens. It is a benign basal cell papilloma with hyperkeratosis and pigmentation. DPN may be diagnosed as melanoma because of cellular pleomorphism and deep dermal infiltration, but the pushing margins, often mild atypia, and lack of mitotic activity help to distinguish it from melanoma. It is practically impossible to diagnose pigmented basal cell carcinoma, which mimics nodular malignant melanoma, except by simple excision and histology. If it is melanoma, a wide reexcision must be done. Hemangioma, especially if thrombosed or bleeding, may be difficult to distinguish from nodular or superficial spreading melanoma except by excision biopsy. Tufted angioma (benign) may be confused with Kaposi's sarcoma or low-grade angiosarcoma, but not with melanoma. Onset is usually before age 5, and the neck, upper chest, and shoulder are frequent sites. Lesions appear as dull-red, mottled macules, 2 to 5 cm in size. Tightly packed capillaries occur in the dermis in ovoid tufts of hypertrophied endothelial cells. Finally, it is obvious that seborrheic keratosis is the most common and difficult lesion to differentiate from melanoma, except for pigmented basal cell carcinoma.

474. The answer is B. *(Wilson, 12/e. pp 1618–1620.)* Tamoxifen, a nonsteroidal antiestrogen that blocks binding of estrogen to the estrogen receptor, was once used as palliative treatment for postmenopausal women with advanced breast cancer but is now widely used in the treatment of selected patients with all stages of breast cancer. It is the best endocrine treatment for advanced breast cancer, but adjuvant tamoxifen therapy also gives increased survival to postmenopausal patients with node-positive disease and to node-negative patients with estrogen-receptor–positive disease. Use of tamoxifen to prevent breast cancer in healthy women is now under clinical investigation.

475. The answer is C. *(Robbins, 4/e. pp 1280–1284, 1288.)* The clinical photograph depicts the presence of the dysplastic nevus syndrome, first described by Dr. Wallace Clark and his coworkers Drs. Mark Greene, David

Elder, and E. Bondi in Philadelphia during the mid 1970s. This valuable finding elucidated the presence of abnormal nevi that are at least a marker for the
development of malignant melanoma. These nevi, while not malignant, have
atypical features compared with those of normal nevi, such as irregular borders, a pink base, and irregular pigmentation. The Leser-Trelat sign refers to
the development of multiple seborrheic keratoses over a short period of time
in older patients who have visceral malignancy, while the basal cell nevus
syndrome is dominantly inherited with the association of numerous basal cell
carcinomas forming throughout life, bifid ribs, keratocysts of the mandible,
unusual facies, and abnormalities of the central nervous system and reproductive system. A familial occurrence of dysplastic nevus syndrome with
basal cell nevus syndrome was elucidated at the 1985 meeting of the Inter-
national Academy of Pathologists by Elliot Foucar. The leopard syndrome
refers to multiple flat lentigines that are not premalignant for melanoma, in
addition to cardiac abnormalities and ocular hypertelorism. Recent studies
have shown that the dysplastic nevus syndrome is not only familial, but may
be sporadic in about 6 percent of the general population. The risk of developing melanoma in the dysplastic nevus familial situation is greatly increased
over that in the general population. It has been stated that patients with dysplastic nevi belonging to a kindred with dysplastic nevus and familial malignant melanoma have a 100-fold risk of developing malignant melanoma over
their entire lifetime.

476. The answer is B. *(Robbins, 4/e. p 1202.)* Gynecomastia is enlargement
of the male breast with marked hyperplasia of duct epithelium and proliferation of periductal connective tissue. No lobular or acinar tissue exists. Gynecomastia often occurs in response to hyperestrinism and may be found with
functioning testicular tumors such as Leydig (interstitial) cell or, rarely, Sertoli cell tumors. The major cause of hyperestrinism in the male is cirrhosis
because of deficient breakdown of estrogenic substances by the damaged
liver. Digitalis therapy occasionally causes gynecomastia, and Klinefelter's
syndrome frequently does so because very reduced circulating androgen results in relative hyperestrinism.

477. The answer is C. *(Robbins, 4/e. pp 1285–1288.)* Fibrous histiocytoma
(dermatofibroma, sclerosing hemangioma) is a benign dermal tumor of fibroblasts and histiocytes, proliferating in cartwheel or storiform pattern, in
which small blood vessels may form a prominent component. Senile (actinic,
solar) keratosis is a premalignant skin lesion with focal atypia of keratinocytes
of the lower layers of the epidermis. There is often a history of chronic exposure to sun, and there is a high incidence in the southern United States.
Other precancerous skin lesions include erythroplasia of Queyrat and the ac-

tive junctional nevus. Keratoacanthoma, a benign tumor, may resemble squamous cell carcinoma both clinically and histologically, but penetration of the dermis never extends deeper than adjacent hair follicles. The lesion is cup-shaped with central keratin; biopsy or excision excludes squamous carcinoma. Bowen's disease is squamous cell carcinoma of the skin in situ. There is no dermal invasion through the basement membrane. The abnormal squamous cells entirely replace the normal epidermis.

478. The answer is A. *(Anderson, 9/e. pp 1741–1745, 1748.)* The most notorious malignant tumor of the breast, presenting a deceptively innocuous histologic and cytologic appearance, is angiosarcoma, with its almost unrecognizable anastomosing clear channels lined by flattened and barely visible endothelial cells. If this combination is seen within unequivocal breast lobules and ducts, the pathologist must suspect angiosarcoma. Well-differentiated adenocarcinoma of the breast (tubular carcinoma) demonstrates a tumor that is rather benign in appearance, with small ducts lined by single and innocuous-appearing epithelial cells. Whereas the primary site of mucinous carcinoma of the breasts (colloid carcinoma), with its "cysts" filled with extracellular mucin and signet-ring cells, presents no problem in diagnosis, biopsies of metastatic lesions will not infrequently show sheets of bland granular cells with pinpoint nuclei resembling granular cell tumor of the skin, a benign lesion. Early intraductal papillary carcinomas have been misdiagnosed at times as benign intraductal papillomas, and the reverse error has also occurred. Infiltrating duct (scirrhous) carcinoma presents no diagnostic problem in either frozen or permanent section analysis for the average pathologist.

479. The answer is D. *(Robbins, 4/e. pp 1193, 1200–1201.)* Carcinoma of the breast still causes about 20 percent of female cancer deaths and is the leading cause of death worldwide in women over 40 years of age. It is difficult to predict survival rate, but the status of the axillary nodes is of major importance since negative nodes suggest 70 to 80 percent 10-year survival. There is a significant decrease in 5-year survival if one to three nodes are positive (only 50 percent), and four or more positive nodes at the time of diagnosis usually mean about 20 percent disease-free survival. Obviously, a large size of involved nodes, invasion of the capsule, and fixation to adjacent tissue adversely affect survival. The histologic type and grade of tumor and its size are important also, but nodal involvement (number and size) is the outstanding factor in prognosis. Unfortunately, more than 20 percent of patients with negative lymph nodes do have recurrences and die within 10 years. Although they are of lesser prognostic importance in breast cancers, high levels of estrogen receptors have a better prognosis than lower levels or none, although the best response to endocrine (antiestrogen) ablation therapy is noted with tumors containing both estrogen and progesterone receptors. Amplified or activated tumor oncogenes, such as the neuoncogene, may be associated with an aggressive tumor and poor prognosis, but this is not yet proved.

480. The answer is D. *(Fitzpatrick, 2/e. pp 360–361. Robbins, 4/e. pp 1198–1199.)* The biopsy shows infiltration of the nipple by large cells with clear cytoplasm, which is diagnostic of Paget's disease. These cells are usually found both singly and in small clusters in the epidermis. Paget's disease is always associated with (in fact begins with) an underlying intraductal carcinoma that extends to infiltrate the skin of nipple and areola. Paget cells may resemble the cells of superficial spreading melanoma, but they are PAS-positive diastase-resistant (mucopolysaccharide- or mucin-positive), unlike melanoma cells. Eczematous dermatitis of the nipples is a major differential diagnosis but is usually bilateral and responds rapidly to topical steroids. Paget's disease should be suspected if "eczema" persists more than 3 weeks with topical therapy. Paget's disease occurs mainly in middle-aged women but is unusual. In Paget's disease of the vulvar-anal-perineal region, there is very rarely underlying carcinoma. Mammary fibromatosis is a rare, benign, spindle cell lesion affecting women in the third decade. Clinically, it may mimic cancer with retraction or dimpling of skin. It should be treated by local excision with wide margins since there is risk of local recurrence.

481. The answer is B. *(Robbins, 4/e. pp 1282–1283.)* Although malignant melanoma of the skin is not as common as squamous and basal cell carcinoma, it is an exceedingly important and somewhat mysterious tumor owing to its often devastating clinical course and occasionally unpredictable behavior. There appear to be strong immune factors that presumably account for some well-documented remissions, lengthy survival after distant metastasis, and rapid growth in renal transplant patients. However, most patients with this form of cancer pursue a course characterized by eventual distant and visceral metastasis, especially if the histologic type is either nodular or superficial spreading. The subtype called *lentigo maligna melanoma,* found in the sun-exposed skin of elderly patients, generally has a much more favorable outlook. The most important predictors of outcome are the level of penetration into the subepidermis and reticular dermis (Clark levels I through V: I, in situ; V, invasion of subcutaneous fat) and the actual depth of invasion, measured in millimeters with an ocular micrometer (Breslow depth). The survival at 5 years is 90 percent if the tumor is Clark I or II and 0.76 mm or less in depth, but survival falls to 40 to 48 percent if the tumor is level III or IV and greater than 1.9 mm in depth. While some melanoma cells may show cytologic pleomorphism, many aggressive melanomas exhibit uniformity and blandness. Recent work has shown that melanomas arising in the region of the shoulder, upper trunk, and back in men behave in an aggressive fashion.

482. The answer is E. *(Robbins, 4/e. p 1199.)* Inflammatory breast carcinoma is often misunderstood because of the qualifying adjective "inflammatory." The term does not refer to the presence of inflammatory cells, abscess, or any special histologic type of breast carcinoma; rather, it refers to more of a clinical phenomenon, in that the breast is swollen, erythematous, and indurated and demonstrates a marked increase in warmth. These changes are caused by widespread lymphatic and vascular permeation within the breast itself and in the deep dermis of the overlying skin by breast carcinoma cells. The clinical induration and erythema are presumably related to lymphatic-vascular blockage by tumor cells; if present, these findings mean a worse prognosis for the patient.

483. The answer is A. *(Robbins, 4/e. pp 199–200, 1137, 1293–1294, 1300–1302.)* The photomicrograph was taken from a patient with superficial spreading malignant melanoma in situ; it shows individual cells resembling Paget's disease invading the upper regions of the epidermis. The basement membrane zone is intact and there are lymphocytes in the underlying dermis. Cells with clear cytoplasm and malignant-appearing nuclei such as shown here resemble those of Paget's disease, from which they must be distinguished. Some cells of mycosis fungoides will resemble this, but they occur in nest formations called Pautrier's abscesses. Metastatic carcinoma can produce lesions that resemble malignant melanoma, but these are problems relating to the dermis. Leukemia-lymphoma infiltrates mainly involve the dermis, although the epidermis may become ulcerated and atrophic. Lupus erythematosus and lichen planus produce subepidermal lymphocytic infiltrates with no involvement of the epidermis itself. Psoriasis produces parakeratosis and elongated rete ridges but no abnormal cells in the epidermis.

484. The answer is E. *(Robbins, 4/e. pp 1187–1191.)* The spectrum of benign breast disease includes fibrocystic disease, which is probably a misnomer; adenosis, both sclerosing and microglandular; intraductal papillomas and papillomatosis; apocrine metaplasia; fibrous stromal hyperplasia; and hyperplasia of the epithelial cells lining the ducts and ductules of the breasts. At one time or another each of the above was considered to be a forerunner of carcinoma; however, with extensive studies in the literature, none of these has been shown to necessarily correlate with a greater risk of developing carcinoma with the exception of epithelial hyperplasia. With any of the features, but especially epithelial hyperplasia, adding a positive family history of breast cancer in a sibling, mother, or maternal aunt markedly increases the risk for developing carcinoma of the breast in the given patient. Owing to the advances and technology of xeromammography, there has been an increased interest in calcifications, which are markers for carcinoma of the breast. These calcifications, however, do not necessarily occur within the cancerous ducts themselves and can be found frequently in either adenosis adjacent to the carcinoma or even in normal breast lobules in the region. Stipple calcification as seen by xeromammography is regarded as an indication for a biopsy of the region by some workers.

485. The answer is D. *(Robbins, 4/e. pp 1298–1299, 1302–1306.)* Patients of either sex in the fourth to sixth decade who develop oral vesicles followed by disseminated bullae are likely to have pemphigus vulgaris, one of the blistering (bullous) dermatoses. The differential diagnosis in this setting is widespread and can include various forms of erythema multiforme (or Stevens-Johnson syndrome in the young) and bullous pemphigoid, as well as pemphigus vulgaris. Common to most bullous dermatoses is the presence of epidermal cell separation, which produces spaces and clefts (acantholysis) that are visible in ordinary tissue sections and specific to location within the epidermis. The bullae may be subcorneal, intraepidermal, suprabasal, or subepidermal, and multiple diseases can be grouped according to acantholysis location. To categorize the type of disease further, direct immunofluorescence testing can be done on a fresh skin lesion, using antibodies to immunoglobulins, fibrin, and complement. Pemphigus vulgaris shows a characteristic "basket-weave" pattern in the epidermis to IgG, IgA is found at the tips of the dermal papillae in dermatitis herpetiformis, and linear bands of IgG and complement are found in the subepidermal zones in bullous pemphigoid, whereas erythema multiforme has no immunofluorescent pattern. In DLE, direct immunofluorescence shows a granular band of immunoglobulin and complement at the dermoepidermal junction (lupus band test), and this may be present in "normal" skin in patients with systemic lupus erythematosus.

486. The answer is B. *(Anderson, 9/e. pp 1730–1731.)* The lesion depicted in the photomicrograph is that of a cellular fibroadenoma, a basically benign neoplasm of the breast. Mueller initially described cystosarcoma phyllodes in 1838 and named it for the resemblance of the lesion to leaves. In older women if the stroma is hypercellular with mitoses and peripheral infiltrative borders, it has the capacity to metastasize. In the adolescent female, cellular stroma of spindle cells with occasional mitoses, such as in this example, may not behave in a malignant fashion as in older women. There is only one documented case of death with dissemination caused by lesions of this type in young girls. Because most lesions like these behave in a benign fashion, conservative but total excision with a small rim of normal tissue surrounding the lesion is all that is necessary in the adolescent.

487. The answer is D. *(Robbins, 4/e. pp 745–746, 1292–1293.)* The photomicrograph demonstrates the presence of Langerhans cells in an infiltrated fashion into the upper dermis and shows the reniform nuclei and crowding characteristic of the disorder previously referred to as a form of *histiocytosis X*. These are now known to be disorders of Langerhans cells, which have surface membrane FC receptors and react with antibodies to thymocyte differentiation antigens (CD1) and ultrastructural granules referred to as *Birbeck granules*. The Letterer-Siwe form arises in children, often in infants, and presents with cutaneous lesions that resemble seborrheic dermatitis (or cradle cap). Often these patients present with fever and otitis media or mastoiditis, which call attention to the disorder. If the disease disseminates it may involve organs of the mononuclear phagocyte system, including the spleen, liver, lymph nodes, bone marrow, and lungs. On x-ray, lesions are reflected by cystic radiolucent areas that can be seen in the skull, pelvis, and long bones. Patients often have anemia and thrombocytopenia, which can contribute to a terminal outcome owing to infections. The term *Langerhans cell granulomatosis* has been offered as an alternative designation to *histiocytosis X, Letterer-Siwe form*. Many infants died from the disorder in years past, but with the use of chemotherapy and improvement of underlying hypoimmunity, there has been a reversal of the death rate. Diabetes insipidus is a fairly common accompaniment.

488. The answer is D. *(Anderson, 9/e. pp 1731–1732, 1737–1739.)* The histologic distinction between benign, cystic intraductal papillomas of the breast and papillary adenocarcinomas is based on multiple criteria. The age of the patient is not of immense importance, since papillomas occur in both younger and older women. Benign papillomas are structured with a complex arrangement of papillary fronds of fibrovascular stalks, covered by one or (usually) two types of cells (epithelial and myoepithelial). Papillary carcinomas are usually of one monotonous cell type and have either no fibrovascular stalks or only a few of them. Papillary carcinomas show a uniform growth of similar-appearing cells with enclosed tubular spaces, with the whole arrangement bridging across the entire lumen at times or simply lining the outer rim of the duct (cribriforming). Peripheral invasion of the stroma, if present at all, makes the diagnosis of carcinoma rather certain. There are lesions in which the differentiation is exceedingly difficult, even in the hands of renowned surgical pathologists. Many competent pathologists understandably prefer to defer the diagnosis on all papillary lesions of the breast on frozen section until well-fixed and optimally prepared permanent sections are available.

489. The answer is B. *(Anderson, 9/e. pp 1769–1771, 1775–1776, 1827.)* Dense lymphocytic infiltration of the skin carries with it a differential diagnosis that includes the five L's: lupus, light, lymphoma, pseudolymphoma, and lymphocytic infiltration of the skin (Jessner). All are characterized by lymphoid hyperplasia of the dermis. Leukemic lymphomas are diagnosed by atypical sheets of lymphoblastic cells with mitoses; lupus erythematosus is characterized by lymphoid infiltration around the follicles and vessels of the dermis. Light eruptions are characterized by a lymphocytic perivascular inflammation on the skin of the face. A difficult differential diagnosis includes lymphocytic infiltration of the skin (Jessner), which often has an increase in dermal mucopolysaccharides that can be demonstrated by alcian blue stains. In urticaria pigmentosa, a localized cutaneous form of mastocytosis that affects mainly children, there is infiltration of mast cells in the upper and middle dermis.

490–494. The answers are: 490-B, 491-C, 492-E, 493-A, 494-A. *(Anderson, 9/e. pp 1757, 1759–1760, 1762–1763, 1772–1774, 1794–1795.)* Acanthosis, or thickening of the epidermis, through hyperplasia of the malpighian layer often occurs with hyperkeratosis, but not always. Although four of the listed lesions are acanthotic, pemphigus vulgaris is acantholytic with loss of intercellular bridges (desmosomes). This type of intraepidermal vesiculation is seen in the bullae of pemphigus vulgaris; cleavage is just above the basal layer. Biopsy and immunofluorescence are necessary for diagnosis of pemphigus.

Psoriasis occurs in up to 2 percent of the population in Western countries. It is a hereditary skin disease with silver-white, scaling plaques often in sites of repeated trauma. Removal of scale results in minute drops of blood (Auspitz sign). Abnormalities of the nails are found in 25 percent of patients, especially in those with arthritis, and include pitting and yellow-brown "oil spots" under the nail. Histologically, there is marked epidermal thickening and thinning with elongation of rete ridges, parakeratotic hyperkeratosis (nuclei retained in the stratum corneum), and increased mitosis of keratinocytes and other cells above the basal layer. Polymorphonuclear neutrophils (PMNs) form the microabscesses of Munro in the stratum corneum of the epidermis.

Lichen planus is an acute or chronic inflammation of the skin and mucous membranes characterized by flat-topped, pruritic, purple papules on the skin and white oral papules. Histologically, lesions show acanthosis with elongated, saw-toothed rete ridges and liquefaction degeneration of the basal layer, often with necrotic basal cells in the papillary dermis, which form colloid or Civatte bodies. There is usually a bandlike lymphocytic infiltrate along the dermoepidermal junction.

Verruca vulgaris, the common wart, is one of the human papillomavirus (HPV 1, 2, 3, 4) infections of the papovavirus group. It may occur anywhere but most commonly appears on the hands and fingers of schoolchildren as firm 1- to 10-mm papules. Histologically, the lesion shows a papillary acanthosis and cells of the stratum granulosum often display perinuclear vacuoles (koilocytosis). Intranuclear viral particles are seen by EM. A characteristic finding is of "reddish-brown" dots (thrombosed capillary loops) seen with a hand lens on the surface.

Acanthosis nigricans occurs most typically in flexures (axilla, groin, ano-genital region) and is usually associated with benign or malignant conditions. The juvenile type is autosomal dominant with variable penetrance and occurs usually in association with obesity or endocrine disorders. The adult type (about 20 percent of all cases) often occurs with occult adenocarcinoma (usually gastric) but has occurred with oral contraceptive use. Folding of a hyperkeratotic epidermis with basal layer darkened with melanin is characteristic of acanthosis nigricans.

495–497. The answers are: 495-E, 496-D, 497-B. *(Robbins, 4/e. pp 1188–1189, 1190–1191, 1194–1195.)* Diseases of the breast that are often painful include galactocele, duct ectasia, and fibrocystic disease. Infiltrating ductal carcinoma rarely causes pain but is likely to produce scirrhous tumors causing a firm or hard mass.

Cystosarcoma phyllodes may be either benign or malignant and has a cellular myxoid stroma in which osteoid or chondroid foci may appear. It forms a large, lobulated, and cystic lesion and malignant change is accompanied by rapid increase in size. Metastases occur only in about 15 percent of cases.

Sclerosing adenosis is benign, does not predispose to carcinoma, is often unilateral, and arises in the upper outer quadrant. It displays clinical and histologic features difficult to distinguish from carcinoma.

None of these three lesions tends to be bilateral—unlike both lobular carcinoma and fibrocystic disease.

498–500. The answers are: 498-C, 499-B, 500-A. *(Anderson, 9/e. p 549. Robbins, 4/e. pp 436–438.)* Marasmus is caused by marked deficiency in total caloric intake, including proteins, carbohydrates, lipids, vitamins, and minerals. Kwashiorkor is linked to marked protein deficiency with adequate or high carbohydrate intake. There are sometimes intermediate forms, or combinations, of these two predominantly childhood diseases. In severe kwashiorkor or marasmus, thymic atrophy occurs with reduction in number and function of circulating T cells. B-cell function (immunoglobulin production) is also depressed, so that these children are highly vulnerable to infections. Dermatoses, characterized by pigment changes and desquamation, are pathognomonic of kwashiorkor. Inelastic wrinkled skin, due to loss of subcutaneous fat, is striking in marasmus.

Bibliography

Anderson WA, Kissane JM (eds): *Pathology,* 9/e. St. Louis, CV Mosby, 1989.

Bullough PG, Vigorita VJ: *Atlas of Orthopaedic Pathology: With Clinical and Radiologic Correlations.* New York, Gower Medical, 1984.

Fitzpatrick TB, et al: *Color Atlas and Synopsis of Clinical Dermatology,* 2/e. New York, McGraw-Hill, 1992.

Graves HCB, et al: Postcoital detection of a male-specific semen protein. *N Engl J Med* 312:338, 1985.

Grizzle WE, Dunlap N: Cushing's syndrome: Diagnosis of the atypical patient. *Arch Pathol Lab Med* 113:727–728, 1989.

Henry JB, et al (eds): *Clinical Diagnosis and Management by Laboratory Methods,* 18/e. Philadelphia, WB Saunders, 1991.

Koss LG: *Diagnostic Cytology and Its Histopathologic Bases,* 3/e. Philadelphia, JB Lippincott, 1979.

Morris JG, et al: Cholera and other vibrioses in the United States, *N Engl J Med* 312:343, 1985.

Ordóñez NG: The immunohistochemical diagnosis of mesothelioma: Differentiation of mesothelioma and lung adenocarcinoma. *Am J Surg Pathol* 13:276–291, 1989.

Peterson WL: *Helicobacter pylori* and peptic ulcer disease. *N Engl J Med* 324:1043–1048, 1991.

Reichert GM, et al: Special topic review. Autopsy pathology in acquired immune deficiency syndrome. *Am J Pathol* 112:357, 1983.

Richart RM: Causes and management of cervical intraepithelial neoplasia. *Cancer* 60:1951–1959, 1987.

Robbins SL, Cotran RS: *Pathologic Basis of Disease,* 4/e. Philadelphia, WB Saunders, 1989.

Rosai J: *Ackerman's Surgical Pathology,* 7/e. St. Louis, CV Mosby, 1989.

Rose BD: *Pathophysiology of Renal Disease,* 2/e. New York: McGraw-Hill, 1987.

Schwartz WB, Wolfe HJ, Pauker SG: Pathology and probabilities: A new approach to interpreting and reporting biopsies. *N Engl J Med* 305:917, 1981.

Takahashi M: *Color Atlas of Cancer Cytology,* 2/e. Tokyo, Igaku-Shoin, 1982.

Tam R: Culture-independent diagnosis of *Chlamydia trachomatis* using monoclonal antibodies. *N Engl J Med* 310:1146, 1984.

Williams WJ, et al: *Hematology,* 4/e. New York, McGraw-Hill, 1990.

Wilson JD, et al (eds): *Harrison's Principles of Internal Medicine,* 12/e. New York, McGraw-Hill, 1991.

MOTOROLA
Software Company